Integrated Quality Management

The Key to Improving Nursing Care Quality

Integrated Quality Management

The Key to Improving Nursing Care Quality

Marylane Wade Koch, RN, MSN, CNAA, CPHQ
Administrator of Alternative Delivery Systems
Methodist Health Systems
Executive Director
Methodist Home Care Services
Methodist Health Systems
Memphis, Tennessee

Terrye Maclin Fairly, RN, BSN
Home Care Consultant
Alpha Medical Incorporated
Chattanooga, Tennessee

Illustrated

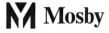

St. Louis Baltimore Boston Chicago London Philadelphia Sydney Toronto

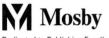

Mosby
Dedicated to Publishing Excellence

Executive Editor: N. Darlene Como
Associate Developmental Editor: Brigitte Pocta
Project Manager: John Rogers
Production Editor: Chris Murphy
Designer: Julie Taugner

FIRST EDITION
Copyright © 1993 by Mosby–Year Book, Inc.

All rights reserved. No part of this publication may be reproduced, stored in a retrieval system, or transmitted, in any form or by any means, electronic, mechanical, photocopying, recording, or otherwise, without prior written permission from the publisher.

Permission to photocopy or reproduce solely for internal or personal use is permitted for libraries or other users registered with the Copyright Clearance Center, provided that the base fee of $4.00 per chapter plus $.10 per page is paid directly to the Copyright Clearance Center, 27 Congress Street, Salem, MA 01970. This consent does not extend to other kinds of copying, such as copying for general distribution, for advertising or promotional purposes, for creating new collected works, or for resale.

Printed in the United States of America

Mosby–Year Book, Inc.
11830 Westline Industrial Drive
St. Louis, Missouri 63146

Library of Congress Cataloging-in-Publication Data
Koch, Marylane Wade.
   Integrated quality management :   the key to improving nursing care quality /   Marylane Wade Koch, Terrye Maclin Fairly. -- 1st ed.
      p.   cm.
   Includes bibliographical references and index.
   ISBN 0-8016-7476-X
   1. Nursing--Quality control.   2. Total quality management.
   I. Fairly, Terrye Maclin.   II. Title.
   [DNLM: 1. Nursing Care–organization & administration. 2. Quality Assurance, Health Care.   WY 100 K76i]
   RT85.5.K6   1993
   362.1'73'0685--dc20
   DNLM/DLC
   for Library of Congress   92-49261
                                                                                       CIP

93 94 95 96 97 CA / MY 9 8 7 6 5 4 3 2 1

Contributors

Sandra S. Bassett, RN, MS, CPHQ
Corporate Director of Quality Improvement
Methodist Health Systems
Memphis, Tennessee

Deborah G. Nance, RN, CPHQ
Director of Professional Services
Regional Health Care Division
Methodist Health Systems
Memphis, Tennessee

To

My husband Rob
who, as a professional peer,
shared the glory and frustrations
of creating a new paradigm.

My parents,
William Doyle and Lottie,
for teaching me to value improvement;
brothers Les and Bill for encouragement.

Jan Biggs Featherstone, Sue Morrisson,
Margaret Page, and Kathryn Skinner
for enduring friendship throughout this process.

My cat, Grace-Anne, my constant companion for 16 years.

And to God, for all the above.

Marylane Wade Koch

God for all gifts and opportunities.

In memory of my father, Gerald E. Maclin

My mother, Margie Bray Maclin,
for teaching me to persevere.

My son, Alexander McKay Fairly, IV, "Mac,"
for giving me many reasons to persevere.

Alexander McKay Fairly, III, "Alex,"
for support and encouragement.

Paul D'Encarnacao, my mentor

Terrye Maclin Fairly

Foreword

AMONG the items I treasure is an old, yellowing copy of an article written by psychiatrist Karl Menninger and published in the Summer 1954 issue of the *Menninger Quarterly*. In this article, Dr. Menninger writes: "Time was when a hospital was a place in which to die. It was not a place of mercy and of healing, but one of endurance, charity, and pity. But the meaning of the modern hospital is quite different. It is no longer an asylum, no longer a pest house, no longer a hotel on the way to God. It is a beacon, a lighthouse—and for all its scenes of suffering—a place of joy. It is a place to which people come, not to die, but to cease dying—a place in which to get well. Temporary refuge it may be and, in another sense from the original, truly a 'hotel of God,' a way station—but not one on the way to death, rather a 'resting place' on the way to life."

If this is the mission—the goal—then it also is the measuring stick of the success of the hospital.

❖ A TIME OF TRANSITION

Few could argue with the proposition that the health care "industry" is in transition: (1) *financially*—from a method that gave individual provider, fee-for-service based reimbursement, to one that favors collective, prepaid managed care; (2) *organizationally*—from a loose, eclectic network of free-standing institutions, agencies, and professionals, to large, multipurpose corporations competing for ever-increasing shares of the market; and (3) *methodologically*—from a system of acute, inpatient, institution-based care, to a system of subacute, outpatient, community-based care.

Hospitals, the traditional backbone of American health care, are in transition, and they are operating in a society that itself is in transition—culturally, morally, and technologically. A pervasive sense of transition breeds skepticism. As institutions, methods, and mores are challenged and changed, stability is undermined, and people lose faith in the constancy of the values, norms, and authorities that shaped the past. The result is a general tendency to distrust, question, and even debunk the authority, purpose, and intentions of organizations and institutions—especially those vital to the public well-being. Moreover, the development of large, collective systems of care delivery inhibits familiarity with persons and even traditions that are basic to the fiduciary relationship, all of which adds to personal withdrawal and alienation. Fear of large-scale institutions adumbrates on those who represent them (administrators, physicians, nurses, and so on). Thus individuals in these positions are required to "prove" themselves constantly because the institutions they represent no longer are deemed trustworthy.

The one constant guaranteeing status and representing success is money. The monetization of status, the equation of worth or value with income, further inhibits recognition of those aspects of professional life/status (commitment, ethical standards, presence, judgment, concern for the social good) that, though not amenable to such quantitative analysis, generally tend to inspire trust and confidence. To illustrate, the word "professional" today is generally used as an antonym for "amateur." A professional is paid; an amateur is not. The more a professional is paid, the "better" professional he or she is perceived to be. In this manner, merit is equated with income, and the punk rock musician who earns $20 million a year is esteemed more highly than the college professor who earns $35,000 a year. Thus social utility becomes secondary to financial gain, which, in turn, sparks fears that professionals will exploit the public to augment their own incomes.

❖ QUALITY, COST, AND OUTCOMES

The problems of society-in-transition are manifest in the health care sector and "concern about quality" is emerging as *the* issue of the decade: the Joint Commission on Accreditation of Healthcare Organizations (JCAHO) included some outcome criteria the last few years; Congress has empowered Peer Review Organizations (PROs) to deny payment to institutions that deliver substandard care; and the media highlight instances of "mismanaged" care. The implications and impact of concern about—and the development of measurements of—quality care are astounding, particularly in light of the ambiguity of the term itself. To begin, does "quality" deal with safety or with amenities? Or with both? Does it consist of *satisfying* the customer or of providing what the patient *needs*—by no means equable measures.

In 1991 the Chairman and Chief Executive Officer of the Prudential Insurance Company of America, Robert C. Winters, keynoted what the JCAHO has called a "landmark" conference, "Cornerstones of Healthcare in the 1990s: Forging a Framework of Excellence." He began his speech with a story: "Recently," Winters said, "a Florida man had the misfortune to step on a splinter. He went to a local hospital to have it removed. He almost had to be rehospitalized when he got the bill: $3,700. That's some set of tweezers!"

❖ THIRTY PERCENT OF CARE IS UNNECESSARY?

Citing Winslow et al. in their 1988 study published in the *New England Journal of Medicine,* Winters quoted the following statistics: 65% of carotid endarterectomies were questionable; 56% of the indications for Medicare-reimbursed pacemaker implantations were either ambiguous or nonexistent . . . and as much as 30% of the medical services delivered in the United States "may be unnecessary, ineffective, or inappropriate."

According to Winters, "physicians control the market and their decisions account for 75 percent of the costs . . . Some people get angry when you suggest that individuals other than physicians should have a voice in deciding what treatments are prescribed . . . Yet, how many of us are getting our money's worth? At the Prudential, we have invested $300 million in developing a national managed care network that will influence prices and treatments. CIGNA, AETNA, Travelers, Metropolitan, Humana, and Kaiser are all doing much the same. Insurance companies are in a whole new business. We don't just write the checks anymore. We manage care. We approve providers, negotiate reimbursement, and screen hospitals. Our goal is to assess the quality and appropriateness of care."

❖ THE PUBLIC: WE'VE GOT TO START SOMEWHERE

Professionals' battles over the validity of measurement data won't be allowed to stop the march toward paying for patient outcomes rather than health care's process. Winters drove home the message from a recent Pennsylvania Health Care Cost Containment Council study: "A quarter of all stroke patients in one hospital died, while in a nearby hospital no stroke patients died. Now some people look at these numbers and call them meaningless . . . That data right now may not take all factors into account. But we've got to start somewhere. The Pennsylvania study found extraordinary differences among hospitals on price and success rates."

And "start," they (and we?) are: in July 1990 nine major payors met with the Managed Health Care Association and InterStudy to design a strategy for outcomes research. Moreover, the Feds aren't lagging far behind. The top priority for the newly founded (and underfunded) Federal Agency for Health Care Policy and Research is the development of medical practice guidelines. Many medical specialty groups have published practice parameters . . . and a hospital quality index—or *Consumers' Guide*—was published in 1992.

❖ JCAHO: PERFORMANCE DATA COMES FIRST

Dr. Dennis O'Leary, president of JCAHO, summed up the conferees' growing consensus on comprehensively tracking providers' care effectiveness in these ways: ". . . Much of our discussion . . . has addressed different aspects of what I will call the 'new evaluation tools' because that's what they really are: standards or guidelines, performance measures, and large, new databases . . . The fact of the matter is that we must look at patient outcomes at different steps along the way. If the ultimate functional outcome is death, that's a little bit late. There are a variety of other intermediate measurement points about which we need information and for which we should have the ability to hold somebody accountable, if only to ask that previous performance be improved in the future.

"Not surprisingly, there seems to be a continuing comfort level with structural standards and structural measures. These include board certification or training that serves as a proxy for likely good performances. As performance data become increasingly available, we may eventually wake up to find out, for instance, that professional training and board certification don't make a large amount of difference. Quite clearly the discomforts of the future are likely to revolve around being willing to acknowledge good performance without requiring that the performer have various tickets as proof of competence. No one disagreed that physicians and other practitioner groups must be intimately involved in development of performance measures and clinical standards . . . Interestingly, and I think reassuringly, there was almost universal agreement that unnecessary and/or ineffective care should not be paid for . . . ."

❖ EVERYBODY'S BUSINESS: TOTAL QUALITY MANAGEMENT

Moreover, Dr. O'Leary continued: "Organizations will be using performance measures, they will be applying clinical standards and practice guidelines, and they will be engaging in continuous quality improvement efforts . . . the rational system of tomorrow will be a standards-based system, but one that progressively emphasizes performance over structural requirements . . . This system will inherently say that one of the important jobs that must get done is to measure and monitor performance. Thus there will clearly be a place for data—data that derives from good performance measures, data that professionals can believe . . . these databases will be crucial because isolated and fragmentary data, particularly in the case of small providers, of which there are many, will be of little use to provider or purchaser . . . ."

Dr. O'Leary concluded: "The Washington bureaucracy is taking a hard-nosed posture. 'Yes,' they tell us, 'we understand that the methods we are using today are not very good, but we intend to use them until something better comes along.' That mentality is pervasive, and it has further raised the stakes. So the name of the game, in a very real sense, is to prudently but expeditiously build a better mousetrap. . . ."

Integrated Quality Management: The Key to Improving Nursing Care Quality offers nursing leaders a practical tool—one of Dr. O'Leary's "better mousetraps"—for integrating quality assessment and improvement into everyday practice. Marylane Wade Koch and Terrye Maclin Fairly are to be commended for clearly and concisely addressing a complex subject.

Leah Curtin, ScD, RN, FAAN
Editor
Nursing Management
August 1992

Preface

IN the 1940s and 1950s health care technology and the discovery of antibiotics led to the proliferation of hospitals and health care delivery. In the 1960s health care access was improved by creation of Medicare and Medicaid, but costs also increased, with the federal government paying the greatest portion of the costs. By the 1970s the government applied regulatory approaches to attempt cost control, and in the 1980s these efforts accelerated. In the 1990s quality, as well as cost and access, became health care's major focus.

Health care delivery today is influenced by multiple factors. There is an ever-increasing number of elderly persons whose primary health care coverage is Medicare. Indigent care is assumed by state-supported Medicaid. Cost for that care continues to escalate while demands for quality and scrutiny of care provided are also increasing. Growing numbers of the chronically ill are living longer. There is also a greater volume of individuals who are uninsured by private insurance yet ineligible for Medicare and Medicaid.

Future trends mandate that high quality, cost-efficient care will be key to the survival of any health care provider. Even today some third-party payors reward providers with preferred contracts, based on positive patient care outcomes. The goal for health care providers is cost management with greater emphasis on quality approaches.

Health care was once assumed to be safe and of high quality. The malpractice crisis of the 1970s was the first indication that "assuming quality" was invalid. With the pressure to manage costs and protect and/or increase market share, progressive health care entities began adopting components of the industrial model of quality and developed similar quality programs. In particular, continuous quality improvement (CQI) and total quality management (TQM) are being implemented in health care settings throughout the United States. CQI and TQM share a management philosophy that enlists every associate or employee of an organization to improve processes through an interdisciplinary "team" approach. As part of improving quality, resources are better managed, and costs are decreased. Such integrated quality management is an essential component of health care continuous quality improvement (CQI) processes. This book illustrates a model for integrating the quality management processes of infection control, utilization management, risk and safety management, and quality assessment into CQI for improved patient care outcomes.

Chapter 1 describes the evolution of quality management and introduces the processes of integrated quality management into CQI. The goals of quality management are defined. Influences that have brought quality to the forefront, such as the media, consumerism, regulation, and reimbursement are discussed. Nursing practice implications are introduced. Chapter 2 describes the concept of synergy in integrated quality management and the implications for today's nursing professional.

Chapter 3 reviews the history of the industrial quality control model and describes the major leaders and their philosophies. A history of health care quality management is then given, and comparisons are drawn between the two. Chapter 4 describes the historical evolution of regulations that affect the individual processes of integrated quality management.

Chapters 5, 6, 7, and 8 give more details of specific processes in integrated quality management. Chapter 9 defines integration and presents Neuman's Systems Model as a conceptual framework for the integrated quality management model. The use of the cause-and-effect diagram, or "fishbone," is introduced as a quality management tool for proactive patient care planning in professional nursing practice.

Chapter 10 describes the necessity and advantages of collaborative practice in integrated quality management. It gives strategies and examples of collaborative quality management for nurses. The opportunity for improved patient care outcomes through interdisciplinary quality improvement teams is explored.

Chapters 11, 12, 13, and 14 offer applications of integrated quality management in various health care settings such as acute care, home care, long-term care, and ambulatory care. Finally, Chapter 15 looks at the future of integrated quality management with discussion of implications for nursing research, ethics, increased technology, and the Nursing Agenda for Health Care Reform.

The authors believe that integrated quality management has great potential for demonstrating the value of professional nursing to the many customers of health care. Some of the benefits to nursing include improved communication, interdisciplinary collaboration and sharing, more coordinated care, and increased visibility for the practicing nurse. Proactive problem solving through integrated quality management means improved patient care outcomes. The end result is better health care with better use of resources and empowerment of professional nurses.

We are especially grateful for the opportunity to publish this book with the patience and diligent editorial assistance of Darlene Como and Brigitte Pocta. We thank Dr. Sylvia Price for her encouragement and mentoring in professional development. We must thank our friends and family for their willingness to allow the time needed for this endeavor. Special thanks to Sandra Bassett for her leadership and coaching as a quality professional peer.

Join us as we explore where nursing has been and where it can go through synergistic integrated quality management. Let's get started. . .there is no time like the present to start shaping the future.

Marylane Wade Koch
Terrye Maclin Fairly

Contents

1

Introduction to Quality Management, 1

2

Processes of Quality Management, 12

3

Quality Management in Business and Health Care, 22

4

Regulatory Influences on Quality Management, 44

5

Quality Assurance/Quality Improvement, 56
Sandra S. Bassett

6

Utilization Management, 73

7

Quality Management in Risk Management and Safety, 90
Terrye Maclin Fairly
Deborah G. Nance

8
Quality Management and Infection Control, 111

9
Integration of Quality Management Processes, 121

10
Implications for Collaborative Practice with Other Disciplines, 138

11
Quality Management in Acute Care, 158

12
Quality Management in Ambulatory Care, 168

13
Quality Management in Home Health Care, 184

14
Quality Management in Long-Term Care, 196

15
The Future of Quality Management: Issues and Trends, 209

Glossary, 225

Appendix A
Integrated Quality Management Tools, 228

Appendix B

Case Studies, 234

Appendix C

National Demonstration Project on Quality Improvement in Health Care, 242

Appendix D

Bibliography, 248

CHAPTER 1

Introduction to Quality Management

THE U.S. health care system moved from the focus of access to health care services in the 1970s to cost containment for care in the 1980s. This has been the prevailing national health care issue in the past decade as demonstrated by the introduction of the federal Prospective Payment System (PPS), which uses a series of diagnostic related groups (DRGs) to determine a hospital's reimbursement for care provided to Medicare patients. Changes in payment methodology created changes in payor attitudes, resulting in alternatives to traditional health care delivery. The system began to restructure. The emergence of alternative delivery systems became the trend. Outpatient services, often considered uncovered for reimbursement in the 1970s, became the preferred alternative in the 1980s. Home care, long-term care, and outpatient services were less expensive ways to deliver some types of health care. The balance of power in health care shifted from the provider to the consumer, mainly third-party payors such as the federal government, businesses, and insurers.

The 1990s marked a new era of focused interest in health care: quality. The question of the consumer is, "Can quality health care be delivered at cost efficient prices?" The challenge to the provider is delivery of quality health care in the most appropriate setting at reasonable cost. As the public becomes more educated, the importance of defining "quality" has come to the forefront. Health care professionals must rise to this challenge by developing and implementing a process that manages the multifaceted issues inherent in quality care.

Although the business industry has already instituted quality control programs, health care facilities have been slow to respond in this area. With the many pressures placed on health care providers in the 1990s, the time has come to implement an integrated quality management process. This chapter defines the components and goals of such a process with the many implications for nursing practice.

❖ DEFINITION OF QUALITY MANAGEMENT
Evolution of Individual Components

Modern quality management is a way of looking at the process of production. First used in industry, it includes concepts such as processes of production, insights into the nature of quality with both successes and failures, and methodology used to plan, improve, and control quality. Each person in the organization is part of a process. The job of each person is to work with others, add value to the product, and pass it on to the customer. The worker is considered the customer, processor, and supplier.[1]

Health care has adopted a similar model for quality management. To address the quality of health care services provided today, administrators must use quality assessment and improvement, utilization management, risk management, safety management, and infection control approaches to improve the "product." Quality improvement is often used synonymously with quality management. This book will use quality management as the more global concept. This philosophy includes clinical components such as quality assessment, infection control, utilization management, and risk and safety management, since the product is health care services.

It also includes quality improvement, which builds on the strengths of quality assurance/assessment (QA) and addresses the weaknesses of QA.[4] In retrospect, Dennis O'Leary of the Joint Commission for Accreditation of Healthcare Organizations (JCAHO) states that quality assurance was an "unfortunate semantic selection," because quality cannot be assured but only improved. Quality can be assessed, so the terminology preferred by the JCAHO in the 1992 standards is quality assessment and improvement.[3]

Most health care agencies have quality assurance processes in place. Quality assurance, now known as quality assessment, provides systematic monitoring and evaluating of patient care delivery. Trends indicating problem areas are determined and activities put in place to resolve the defined problems. Follow-up is necessary to be sure no new concerns have appeared and corrective actions have been effective.

The role of infection control has been established in some dedicated function for many years in most health care facilities. Infection control programs are designed to identify and prevent the spread of infection in the health care setting and community. If the environment is free of infectious contaminants, patients, visitors, and staff can be safe from unnecessary exposure to disease. This component of quality management is certainly a basic but crucial one.

Much attention has focused on utilization management in the past decade. Although utilization review was first required in the Social Security Amendments of 1965, little action was taken. In 1980 JCAHO established the first utilization review standard to look at appropriate levels of care for certain patient health care problems. Utilization management now has a specific place in quality management. This concern is reflected in the national interest in hospital average length of stay (ALOS), a measurement used in assigning federal dollars based on DRGs. Each day of health care resources spent inappropriately affects the overall ability of the health care system to provide quality services.

A more recent emphasis is risk management and safety. This function minimizes the exposure of the provider through risk identification and decreased adverse outcomes to the consumer and provider staff. Liability is associated with professional malpractice exposure of physicians, nurses, and other staff like physical therapists and pharmacists; workman's compensation; and property and causality exposure associated with plant and equipment maintenance. Risk management standards were introduced into the 1990 JCAHO standards for health care agencies seeking accreditation.

Integration into Quality Management

What is often missing in even the most sophisticated organizations is the integration of all quality management components. JCAHO has as its focus "continuous quality improvement (CQI)." Some organizations call their quality improvement program Total Quality Management (TQM). Whatever the term used, the goal is the same: to expand traditional quality processes to include all clinical, administrative, and support functions to improve the quality of health care services.

> ## Quality Management Questions
>
> - Where and how are the quality functions organized?
> - Are the functions sharing information?
> - What are the processes by which communication is promoted?
> - Does the organizational reporting structure facilitate coordination?
> - Is the system designed to support integration of the components?
> - Is there duplication in functional roles?
> - Are clinical, support, and administrative departments performing the quality management process in a comprehensive, efficient manner?
> - Are professional care givers included in the quality assessment and improvement process?

Senior management must take the lead in assessing the agency's progress toward integrated quality management. They must ask several questions and answer them honestly (see box above). These questions are important as administration defines the organization's quality assessment and improvement plan. Integrating the clinical components of quality management into the daily practice of the professional staff is mandatory if quality improvement is to be demonstrated. The evolving concept of CQI and TQM will be discussed in Chapter 5, entitled "Quality Assurance/Improvement."

Quality management can be used to define both the abstract philosophy and the concrete workings of an integrated program that includes at least, but is not limited to the following (Fig. 1–1):

1. Quality assessment and improvement
2. Infection control
3. Utilization management
4. Risk management/safety

It is believed these areas are so dependent on each other that the whole is enhanced by their integration. The concept of *synergy* is inherent to this process.

Buckminster Fuller, a great American designer, engineer, and architect, expressed this concept well as ". . . the behavior of a whole system unpredicated by the behavior of its components or any subassembly of its components."[2] Webster defined synergism as "the simultaneous action of separate

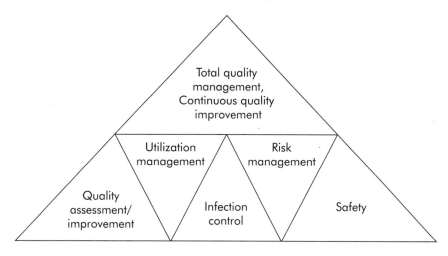

FIGURE 1-1
Integrated quality management.

agencies which, together, have a greater total effect than the sum of their individual effects. . . ."[5] It is this effect that can be achieved by integration of the individual parts of quality management.

The challenge by external parties for health care agencies to review their internal systems forces such a process to the forefront. Most agencies lack such an approach but will find it crucial to survival in the health care industry of the 1990s. Management must adopt a prevailing philosophy that provides the open, honest environment for the quality management process to flourish. Individual departments must disregard "turf" issues and work for the good of the whole system. The quality management process must be part of clinical, administrative, and support services. The CEO must make this philosophy endemic if quality improvement is to take place. The corporate culture must exemplify the belief system that each department is accountable for the quality of care provided to the consumer.

❖ GOALS OF QUALITY MANAGEMENT

The goals of quality management are defined both in comprehensive and specific terms. The goal of providing "high quality care" is often seen in the mission statements of health care agencies, especially hospitals. Quality management strives to create a positive, open, and honest culture that provides health care services judiciously. The process is designed to monitor and trend problems, review organizational processes and services, protect the consumer from adverse outcomes, and guard the agency from loss.

Processes are put in place to decrease and control the spread of infectious disease among staff and patients. Quality management facilitates the opportunities for identification and implementation of quality assessment and improvement. This process is useful in demonstrating agency excellence.

Another goal of quality management is to assist the consumer and provider in maximizing resource management. Financial return to the provider can increase as quality care is demonstrated through accurate documentation, which facilitates reimbursement by payors. A quality reputation can mean satisfaction to the consumer and increased market share to the provider.

A major goal of quality management is education of the consumer and agency staff about what are reasonable and acceptable health care services at affordable prices. The consumer expectations of the appropriate setting for a certain service may differ from the quality manager's perspective. The goal of a safe practice environment for the appropriate level of care needed must be determined. The public may perceive that care is poor if it is not delivered in the location expected and is not provided by a certain level of health care professional. Effective education will help to ease the emotions expressed by both staff and patient as care is given safely with minimal adverse outcomes in alternative settings.

A result of quality management can be increased agency morale as professionals experience providing good quality care. A well-defined and functional quality management process can increase morale of the staff and, in turn, assist with recruitment and retention of qualified staff. Again, the system and consumer will benefit from the quality improvement that results.

❖ INFLUENCES ON QUALITY MANAGEMENT
The Media Emphasis

The focus on health care quality management issues has increased through media attention. A journal rarely completes an issue without giving some attention to health care issues. Women's magazines publish articles on subjects such as how much health care testing should cost and picking a "quality" doctor. Newspapers carry stories on health care costs and quality on a daily basis. Highlights of the many diverse problems in delivering and receiving quality health care are on television programs such as 60 Minutes, 48 Hours, and CNN.

Investigations of health care statistics make excellent sources for sensational stories as the media presents the public with information such as mortality and morbidity rates at specific hospitals. The *Wall Street Journal* addresses health care costs and quality on a consistent basis. *U.S. News and World Report* prints health care stories; a recent one, "Looking Over the Doctor's Shoulder," caused quite a reaction in letters to the editor. Even radio talk shows find an active audience when discussing health care delivery issues.

Consumerism: Client Satisfaction

Consumer satisfaction is paramount in the eyes of the U.S. public. As reimbursed health care dollars decrease, increased market shares must be sought for the agency's survival in a competitive market. With shrinking health care reimbursement, consumer influence is even more crucial. The perceived "quality" of any health care agency will influence the extent to which products and services are bought by the consumer.

Consumers and third-party payors now have a choice and exercise the right to "shop." The "baby boomers" want more control over health care decisions. Consumers are more educated and sophisticated than they were in the past decade. These factors influence and pressure health care facilities to design effective ways to measure and evaluate services.

Consumer groups such as the American Association of Retired Persons (AARP) and business and health coalitions have tremendous power in political issues affecting health care delivery. In recent years, the catastrophic care bill, so long desired by Medicare recipients and the late Senator Claude Pepper, was defeated because of effective lobbying against the act by groups like the AARP. This bill would have provided more health care dollars to fund the needs of the older adult in America, a utilization management issue. However, the Medicare recipients would have incurred additional costs for the coverage.

Regulation and Reimbursement

An economics professor once told his class, "Politics and economics . . . that's what runs the health care industry." This is certainly true in the case of quality management. Only when payment was attached to utilization of resources, as in DRGs, and mandated by the federal government for Medicare recipients did health care providers begin to develop utilization management skills. As malpractice claims became more prevalent and the consumer began to win, risk management became important to help define "quality."

When the Peer Review Organization (PRO) was charged by the federal government with medical record review for appropriateness and quality of care, with monetary sanctions attached, quality management concerns began to grow. The JCAHO came under scrutiny for accrediting facilities that did not maintain quality standards after the survey process was complete. Greater emphasis was placed on ongoing monitoring and evaluating of care through quality assurance programs. The Health Care Financing Administration (HCFA) aligned with JCAHO to receive reports of substandard care in facilities receiving Medicare reimbursement.

Likewise, business and consumer groups began to shop for the "best product at the best price." Again, as providers bargained for comprehensive health care plans with preferred provider contracts, economics and politics came into the decision. The stipulation for the 1990s is quality at reasonable costs.

❖ IMPLICATIONS FOR NURSING PRACTICE

Nurses, as primary managers of care in most health care settings, can benefit greatly through implementing a quality management process. It is nursing that is cited so often in consumer satisfaction surveys as an indicator of quality care. The nurse must practice both the "art" of professional nursing, that of communication, compassion, and interpersonal skill, as well as the "science," the technical skills for care delivery.

The nurse's documentation in nursing notes is vital to quality management. Thorough and accurate documentation is part of the program as utilization management looks at judicious resource consumption. This means the nurse has a direct impact on the reimbursement paid by third-party payors for health care services. The risk management component is apparent as the same accurate documentation protects the nurse and the institution from litigation.

Nurses carry primary responsibility for controlling the spread of infectious disease. Today, major life-threatening infectious diseases still exist in the United States. Antibiotic resistance is increasingly a problem in the pharmacologic treatment of disease. Drug costs continue to soar. Quality management can minimize the risk of exposure of patient and staff to such infectious disease.

Nurses are often responsible for patient and family education. They can be most instrumental in assisting the patient to understand why he is in a given setting to receive his care. Nurses can help manage resources (utilization management) by patient and family teaching before discharge from the setting. Adequate teaching gives the patient the opportunity to accept responsibility for his health and his care. Again, the quality management process has been employed to improve patient care.

Quality management is an excellent way to promote professional practice and demonstrate excellence. This gives nursing an image boost so needed in today's health care environment. Quality management can assist in securing respect and autonomy for the nursing profession.

❖ IMPLICATIONS FOR NURSING ADMINISTRATION

Although industry has strengthened its position through quality management, more health care organizations are demonstrating similar success. In the fall of 1987, 21 health care organizations became participants of the National Demonstration Project on Quality Improvement in Health Care (NDP). The research question for this project was "Can the tools of modern quality improvement with which other industries have achieved breakthroughs in performance help in health care as well?"[1]

Berwick identifies 10 success factors that are evident in any institution that improves quality and reduces quality-related costs. These are of utmost importance to the nursing administrator as the leader of quality management in the practice of professional nursing administration (see box on p. 10).

❖ SUMMARY

The 1990s are sure to be an era in which defining, measuring, and evaluating quality care will be paramount. No longer can individual departments of quality assessment and improvement, infection control, utilization management, and risk management/safety function independently. The changing times demand a synergistic approach that produces a comprehensive positive outcome: quality health care provided in a safe environment by

> ### *Management-Directed Success Factors*
>
> Senior management must:
> - Personally direct the new quality management approach by guiding and serving on a quality leadership council.
> - Apply quality improvement methods to business processes and traditional operating processes.
> - Attend the needs of internal and external customers.
> - Adopt the idea of mandated, annual quality improvement.
> - Develop an infrastructure to identify opportunities to improve and assign responsibility for getting this done.
> - Endorse the concept of planning for quality with those impacted by the plan as participants.
> - Replace empiricism in quality planning with modern quality methodology.
> - Train all members of management in modern quality processes such as quality planning, quality control, and quality improvement.
> - Provide opportunities for the workforce to receive training as well as be active participants in quality management processes.
> - Enlarge the strategic business planning process to include quality goals and a means to meet those goals.
>
> From Berwick DM, Godfrey AB, Roessner J: *Curing health care: new strategies for quality improvement,* San Francisco, 1990, Jossey-Bass.

competent, caring professionals at reasonable cost. The media, regulations, reimbursement guidelines, consumers, and third-party payors will expect and respect integrated quality management.

The corporate culture must be an honest one where quality improves in a systematic fashion. Each department must have individual and collaborative responsibility for implementing the quality management process in both clinical and administrative areas. Senior management must accept accountability for the total implementation of quality improvement.

Nursing's role is primary as the nurse is the closest to the consumer for the most consistent periods of time. The nursing "art" of compassion, caring, and interpersonal relations will complement the "science" of nursing as levels of technical competence will be measured. Nursing can affect reimbursement through appropriate documentation and assessing risk exposure. The quality management process will give nursing the image boost needed in today's controversial environment, promoting autonomy and research in professional practice. This is an area where nurses can make a major positive impact on health care delivery in the 1990s.

REFERENCES

1. Berwick DM, Godfrey AB, and Roessner, J: *Curing health care: new strategies for quality improvement,* San Francisco, 1990, Jossey-Bass.
2. Fuller RF: *Ideas and integrities,* New York, 1963, Collier Books.
3. O'Leary, DS: CQI—a step beyond QA, *Quality Rev Bull,* Jan. 1991.
4. Roberts DM, Schyve PM: From QA to QI: the views and roles of the Joint Commission, *The Quality Letter,* May 1990.
5. *Webster's New World Dictionary of the American Language,* College edition, Cleveland and New York, 1968.

CHAPTER

2

❖

Processes of Quality Management

Quality management is a systematic way to continually improve a product or service. In the quality revolution the question asked by the customer is "How well was it done?" The customer considers a product or service he or she can trust "quality." In the industrial revolution whoever made the most was successful. In today's quality revolution whoever makes the best will win. This is as true for health care service delivery as for any other business.

Management must practice a quality philosophy that encourages the people providing the service to trust each other, work together, and to be creative in service improvement. A major part of delivering quality services is the skill of the people who provide the service. These people must work together effectively to improve the services and delight the customer. The organizational infrastructure must support the continuous quality improvement process.

The principle of synergy is of utmost importance to the manager who implements quality management in the workplace. It is this concept put into practice that empowers a quality management team and makes it work. Webster defines the word "synergy" as "the interaction of discrete agencies or agents such that the total effect is greater than the sum of the individual effects."[6] It is this concept that makes the various processes unique to themselves but more powerful together.

This concept applied effectively in quality improvement teams can guarantee continuous quality improvement in any health care setting. An integrated, synergistic quality management process will be the competitive strength of any health care organization. To understand the potency of synergy in quality management, a thorough understanding of the synergy "concept" is necessary.

❖ CHARACTERISTICS OF SYNERGY

Covey describes synergy as the highest activity of life and considers synergy the essence of principle-centered leadership.[1] In his book, *The Seven Habits of Highly Effective People*, Covey writes that synergy unleashes great power in people as it unifies them in their mutual causes.

Synergy basically means that the whole is greater that the sum of its parts. The relationship that each part has to the other is unique, and differences are valued. In fact, it is the respect for the individual differences of each party that allows the "whole" to build on strengths and compensate for weaknesses. This process is catalytic, unifying each part and empowering the "whole." The result of synergy can be a new and improved alternative: something that was not there before.

Because synergy is a creative process, the participants must have a sense of adventure. There is a spirit of discovery as the "whole" is realized in evolving ways. The participants in synergy must be internally secure because they will have to leave the comfort zone of their individual part to become part of the "whole." Synergy requires each part to be a pathfinder, confronting new territory, as well as the unknown. The reward is new and better possibilities that others may follow.

❖ NATURAL SYNERGY

Covey gives several examples of synergy that occur naturally in our world. When two plants are placed close together in the soil, the roots mingle together and improve the quality of the soil. This allows better growth and nourishment than if each plant had been alone.[1]

Another example of natural synergy is the strength of wood. When two pieces of wood are placed together, they can hold much more weight than either can alone. Again, the concept of synergy demonstrates that $1 + 1 = 3$ or more.

In nursing school, students are taught that certain drugs given in combination provide a better effect. This is synergy in pharmacology: "one drug potentiates (multiplies) the effects of another drug."[3] Basically, a synergistic pharmacologic effect occurs when "two drugs producing the same qualitative effect are combined to produce a greater response than either drug given alone."[7] This is distinguished from an additive effect because synergism produces an effect greater than the sum of the drugs' separate effects.[3] The result may be potentiation of the intensity of the drug's effect or prolongation of its action.

An example of synergy in pharmacology is when ethanol, a central nervous system (CNS) depressant, is combined with barbiturates and tranquilizers. The sedative effect with resulting psychomotor skills impairment is enhanced.[7] Another example of synergism in pharmacology is in the case of certain antibiotics. Co-trimoxazole, a combination of sulfamethoxazole and trimethoprim, is known to have a better effect than either of the two components alone. Alone, the effect is bacteriostatic, whereas together the effect is bacteriocidal.[7]

❖ SOCIAL SYNERGY

The quality revolution requires a philosophy change of leadership. This will produce a social or cultural change in the organization. Quality improvement teams require "social synergy" to produce the continuous improvement of products or services. The nurses providing the health care services must work as an effective team and create improved service delivery through integrated quality management.

To better apply this principle, the example of the family as social synergy is described. The conception of a child is synergistic because two very different individuals, the male and female, unite to form a union in the mother's womb. Again, differences are respected and valued, another important part of the synergy concept. The male and female have physical, social, mental, and emotional differences. These differences, conceived as a child, create a whole new life. Positive aspects to this new "whole" can be an individual who is more giving, less political, more trusting, less defensive, and less adversarial than either of the parents. Synergy can create a new and fulfilling environment.[1]

Another part of social synergy takes place in the arena of communication. For synergy to occur, the parties must have an open mind and appreciate new alternatives. When the process of synergy takes place in the social or communication setting, no one knows how the "whole" will turn out.

There is excitement and adventure. Each party must believe that the "whole" will be significantly better that the parts alone. The results are more insight gained, mutual learning, and momentum created for growth. An example of synergy is the crisis situation where everyone works together despite differences and, for the moment, leaves the ego of self for the good of the whole. There is pride in the finished "whole" when a life is saved or a crisis is resolved. This is social synergy.

As already stated, synergy requires each participant to leave the comfort zone of his or her territory and experience the excitement of synergy. This means having a significant amount of personal security and the integrity of personal principles and values. The person must have a high tolerance for ambiguity because this is often part of synergy as the "whole" is in process. This can be unpleasant if one needs the comfort of structure, certainty, and predictability.

What happens as social synergy takes place through communication? The group becomes close and genuinely tries to understand each person's position. Each develops respect for the other. When differences occur, the attitude is one of "help me understand your point of view as you are a competent and valuable partner in the group." Covey describes the result as nonprotective interaction. Solutions that are better than those originally proposed are produced, and all parties know this. Excitement replaces boredom as high trust and pride in a creative enterprise occurs. A whole that is better than the sum of its parts becomes reality.

❖ ORGANIZATIONAL SYNERGY

As the quality management philosophy is embraced, organizational restructuring may take place. Decentralized decision making is a primary theme as the people closest to the service delivered are empowered to make change. Kanter[2] points out that the point of the present-day organizational restructuring is to achieve synergy. Kanter states that this can be difficult to achieve unless the players are correct and the process is positive. Certain threats to the achievement of synergy in the organization can be confusion, misinformation, loss of energy, emotional leakage, loss of key resources, breakdown of initiative, need for scapegoats, and loss of faith in a leader's ability to deliver as promised.[2]

Competition can be destructive to synergy. Player attitudes actually can subtract rather than add to the "whole." This is true when the participants become more interested in beating their peers than in performing well. Another detrimental effect of competition is depressed performance as attitudes of distrust and suspicion suppress creativity.[2]

Organizational synergy requires sensitivity to the process of change, as well as interest in the needs and concerns of the people involved. Performance standards can be raised as the team builds commitment through shared goals. To have organizational synergy, bonds must be built among the participants. Each party must contribute something to the "whole" and be focused on cooperative and integrated activities. This will add value through enhanced communication and social synergism. Outcomes of organizational synergy are combined expertise, improved efficiency, and a foundation for relational communication.[2]

❖ VALUED DIFFERENCES

The quality management philosophy encourages and values the differences and the uniqueness of the diverse health care team. All people are different in many ways and alike in others. To have true synergy take place, differences must be considered of great value. This may require humility on the part of the participants. Each must recognize his or her own perceptual limitations. Appreciation of the rich resources that differences afford the "whole" must be affirmed. Differences can add understanding and knowledge of reality. Perceptions can be clarified for greater accuracy.

This can be especially powerful when dealing with the negative forces accompanying change and growth. When people are involved in a process, understand and value any different opinions, and own the process, creative solutions can result. New shared goals are set and made possible as the participants become empowered by synergy.[1] The opportunity for improvement of health care services increases when differences are valued and synergy occurs.

❖ QUALITY MANAGEMENT: THE COMPONENTS

The 1990s marks a decade of informed consumerism. Today's consumers demand a high standard of product or service for which they spend their dollars. The power has shifted from the provider to the buyer or customer. More and more, this customer expects a quality service at lower costs. This is especially true in the health care service industry as costs have continued to rise for several decades. The need for a continuous quality improvement process that addresses the monitoring and evaluation of health care services is a must for any agency. An integrated, synergistic quality management program will be the health care agency's competitive edge.

❖ QUALITY ASSESSMENT AND IMPROVEMENT

Quality assessment and improvement (QA/QI) is the systematic monitoring process that identifies opportunities for improvement in patient care delivery, designs ways to improve the service, and continues to evaluate follow-up actions to make certain that improvement occurs. Improvement steps taken are effective. The JCAHO has standards that state that an ongoing quality assessment and improvement process can objectively and systematically monitor and evaluate both the quality and appropriateness of patient care delivery. The process also will provide opportunities to improve care and resolve any identified problems.

This societal commitment evolved from the responsibility that professionals have for self-regulation in society. Health care professionals assume the right of governing themselves by controlling the quality of services provided.[5] In this manner, quality assessment and improvement may serve as the unwritten contract between the health care agency and the public.[4]

Quality assessment and improvement is an integral part of quality management. Some trace its beginnings to 1858, the Crimean War, when Florence Nightingale identified problems and attempted to set certain standards to improve nursing practice. More emphasis was given to the process when the JCAHO began its independent organization to promote quality health care in 1956.

With the establishment of Medicare in 1966, quality assurance, the predecessor of quality assessment and improvement, became more important as a means of maintaining quality of care for Medicare recipients. The JCAHO established a standard for quality assurance in 1980 with revision in 1985. In 1992, the JCAHO standard was named more appropriately "Quality assessment and improvement."

Today, the quality assessment and improvement process is one that almost all health care providers are learning and implementing. This program of ongoing, planned monitoring and evaluation of patient care is a crucial part of integrated quality management.

❖ RISK MANAGEMENT

The risk management (RM) part of quality management demonstrates an ongoing improvement process that determines potential and actual organizational losses. This process identifies the likelihood of organizational loss, estimates the severity of these losses, and equates this to dollars. Risk management is practiced by assessing and improving organizational policy, making decisions, and implementing risk awareness processes. When in place, these processes can avert losses and minimize exposure. The best way to achieve risk management is through risk prevention, or preventing adverse outcomes for the organization, its staff, and its customers.

Risk management has diverse implications in protecting the organization. One method is trending incident reports or occurrence screenings. Others include claims management, contract review, and professional liability programs. Safety and security processes fall under risk management with emphasis on disaster preparation and preventive maintenance programs. Data collection and analysis that can strengthen the risk management process are patient education programs, patient advocacy programs, and patient satisfaction surveys.

Risk management operates individually and collectively with other quality management processes to provide minimal risk in the health care setting so that quality health care is provided in a safe environment. Risk management has a unique role in integrated quality management.

❖ UTILIZATION MANAGEMENT

Utilization management (UM) is the planning, organizing, directing, and controlling of the health care product in a cost-effective manner while maintaining quality of patient care and contributing to the overall goals of the institution as defined by the American Hospital Association. It is an extension of utilization review (UR), the process of evaluating the use of professional medical services, procedures, and facilities against preestablished criteria. The primary process of UR is concurrent review of admission that assures initial and continued hospitalization is needed and that this is the correct level of care for the condition. UM, on the other hand, identifies and improves processes that cause or result in inappropriate utilization of resources and efficient delivery of health care.

Although required by the Social Security amendments of 1965, UM gained credibility in quality management in the 1980s. Historically a retrospective payment system encouraged excessive resource consumption. The hospital was paid by the day and by the tests delivered in the facility. The JCAHO developed the UR Standard in 1980, but the Tax Equity and Fiscal Responsibility Act (TEFRA) in the early 1980s gave emphasis to a prospective payment system, which resulted in DRGs. The Peer Review Organization (PRO) was established by the federal government to monitor health care covered in its budget for appropriate utilization and quality of care. Other factors such as inappropriate scheduling of services that cause delay in treatment also surfaced as UM became part of each facility's quality management process.

UM continues to maintain an active position in most facilities as management strives to maximize the bottom line with more limited resources. Discharge planning and UM must work together to plan appropriate level of care for each patient with reasonable resource consumption. UM is a major player in the integrated quality management process by complementing the other processes.

❖ INFECTION CONTROL

Infection control (IC) is probably the oldest part of quality management. Understanding communicable disease as an illness that is caused by a specific agent or toxic substance is a basic premise to infection control principles. Transmission modes and communicable disease causes are necessary concepts that the health care provider must know to practice in a safe environment.

Certain key factors are necessary for trending and reporting in infection control. The type and scope of surveillance must be determined with certain reports such as nosocomial or clean wound rates generated for use by the quality management practitioner. Prevalence and incidence data can be gleaned through studies with appropriate action and follow-up. Then, ongoing surveillance must take place.

Infection control is a specific and individualized part of the synergistic quality management process. It is often the data from infection control that impacts the other quality management processes. Infection control is unique and necessary to integrated quality management.

❖ QUALITY MANAGEMENT SYNERGY

The processes of quality management are distinct entities that offer much individually. However, when these powerful individual processes are integrated and become synergistic, exciting and innovative alternatives, which were not present initially, occur. Each is related and builds on the strengths of the other. Quality assessment trends are available to risk management or utilization management for improved quality services. Customer satisfaction surveys can be integrated into the quality improvement process. Infection control or safety opportunities become indicators for quality assessment and improvement (QA/QI), and change can take place. It is this integrated synergy that gives strength to the quality management process.

When the professional nursing team understands the unique processes of QA/QI, RM, UM, and IC, synergy automatically takes place to blend and search for better ways to provide quality patient care. The following chapters will define each process in greater detail and give examples of integrated quality management in various health care settings.

❖ SUMMARY

Quality management demands a synergistic culture that empowers quality improvement of health care services in all settings. Synergy is as natural as nature itself. Ecology is an example of the concept because everything is related and dependent on something else in nature. Social interaction and communication can exemplify synergy as each party brings an open mind, differences, and ownership of the "whole" to the process. The more sincere and genuine the participation in the synergistic process, the greater the results and the more commitment to the new creation, the "whole." Teamwork, team building, and unity truly can take place as change and growth occur in the organization through synergy.

The way to provide the appropriate level of quality health care with reasonable resource consumption is through the constant synergy of these quality management processes. Each, though unique and different, empowers the total process and a new "whole" is created as quality improvement of services occurs.

The process of integrated quality management is an excellent way to demonstrate nursing's value and dedication to professional health care delivery and nursing practice. As nurses employ QA/QI, RM, UM, and IC and work together in quality improvement teams, the health care services provided will meet the needs of their customers in all settings. Nurses will directly affect the value society places on quality health care services.

REFERENCES
1. Covey SR: *The seven habits of highly effective people,* New York, 1989, Simon & Schuster.
2. Kanter RM: *When giants learn to dance,* New York, 1989, Simon & Schuster.
3. *Learning about drug interactions, Nursing now series,* Springhouse, Pa, 1984, Springhouse.
4. Phanuef M: *Nursing audit: profile for excellence,* New York, 1972, Appleton-Century-Crofts.
5. Simms LM, Price SA, Ervin NE: *The professional practice of nursing administration,* New York, 1985, John Wiley & Sons.
6. *Webster's New World Dictionary of the American Language,* College edition. Cleveland and New York, 1987.
7. Williams BR, Baer CL: *Essentials of clinical pharmacology in nursing,* Springhouse, Pa, 1990, Springhouse.

CHAPTER

3

❖

Quality Management in Business and Health Care

THE 1990s has "quality" as a buzzword in almost every written work, speech, or conversation. Consumers and third-party payors expect "quality care," with little definition applied. Although quality measurement is new to health care as an industry, other businesses have employed sophisticated methods of quality control for many years. More and more, providers and consumers try to apply the industrial model of measuring quality to the service industry of health care. To compare the two, the reader must understand the history and development of quality control in the business world.

❖ QUALITY MANAGEMENT IN BUSINESS
History of Total Quality Control

The history of modern-day quality control can be traced to Dr. W.E. Shewhart of the Bell Laboratories in the 1930s. Dr. Shewhart developed the control chart and began its application in industry. World War II, however, forced use of the control chart and made it possible for the United States to produce military supplies in large quantities and inexpensively. The quality control standards of that time were called Z-1 Standards. Some think the war was won by quality control and modern statistics application. This information was considered "classified information"[11] (Fig. 3-1).

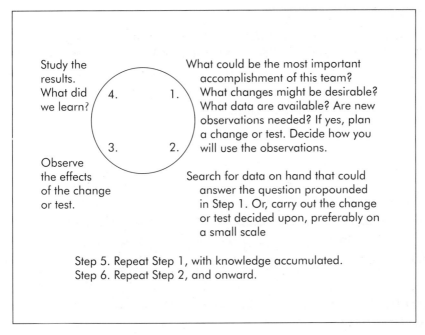

FIGURE 3-1
The Shewhart cycle. (From Deming WE: *Out of the crisis*, Cambridge, Mass, 1986, Massachusetts Institute of Technology.)

England also began applying some quality control statistics (British Standards 600) in 1935 based on E. S. Pearson's work. Britain later adopted the United States' Z-1 Standards.

Japan, devastated by the war, had few industries. The U.S. government, stationed in Japan, was soon annoyed by the inefficiency of the telephone communication system. It found the quality of the equipment to be poor and inconsistent. The United States ordered the Japanese to institute some basic quality control principles and began the education process for this. Modern statistical quality control began in Japan in 1946. Results were good, and Japan went on to become a leader in quality control and quality of goods produced. Several American leaders in quality control made this possible with consultations to Japan in the 1950s. Today the Japanese commitment to quality control is more defined than it is in the United States.

Definitions of Terms: Quality Control

Quality control has been defined narrowly as quality of products or services. The Japanese Industrial Standards define it as, "a system of production methods which economically produces quality goods or services meeting the requirements of consumers."[11] This definition is often combined with "modern" quality control that includes utilization of statistical methodology. In this combination the term used is "statistical quality control."

Others have defined quality control in various ways. Ishikawa, one of the world's foremost authorities on the subject, states, "to practice quality control is to develop, design, produce, and service a product which is economical, most useful, and always satisfactory to the customer."[11] Broadly, one can consider quality control to include everything from quality of human resources such as managers, workers, and executives to quality of the company or its systems.

Leaders in Quality Improvement: Development and Implementation

Dr. W. Edwards Deming. Dr. W. Edwards Deming, PhD. is an internationally known lecturer and consultant who has led many businesses in development and implementation of quality control programs. He has degrees in mathematics, engineering, and physics. In 1946 Dr. Deming established a private practice as a statistical consultant. He became a faculty member at New York University in the business administration graduate program where he taught statistical sampling and quality control.[18]

Deming is best known for his work in Japan, although American companies have sought his wisdom recently in developing quality management in businesses. In 1950 Deming presented an 8-day workshop in Japan on statistical quality control for managers. His outline included how to use the Deming cycle of "Plan, Do, Check, and Action" (PDCA) to improve quality, as well as emphasis on understanding statistical data and process control through control charts.

In recognition for his achievements the Union of Japanese Scientists and Engineers started an Annual Deming Prize for advancement and dependability of a given product.[11] In 1980 the Annual Deming Medal was established by the Metropolitan Section of the American Society for Quality Control. This award was for achievement in application or theory used for improvement in quality and productivity.[6]

What was Deming's message? He consulted from business to business and lecture to lecture explaining to top-level management in America that quality improvement and consequent productivity enhancement would put U.S. businesses in a more competitive position. He explained that failure to manage for the future would result in resource wastes of manpower, materials, and machine time. The new management emphasis would have to be on nurturing long-range plans that would generate new products and services that would keep the company and its employees secure. He charged that American industry was losing competitive strength and creating unemployment because of the failure of the upper leaders to manage.[6]

The solution Deming proposed was dedication to improvement of quality and productivity to secure the needed competitive position. This process would take great education because few schools offered courses on quality improvement. The responsibility for change was on the shoulders of the management team. A long-term commitment to a new philosophy was required: a philosophy that sought quality and productivity improvement.

Deming taught that the key to increased productivity was quality improvement. In his opinion low quality means low productivity. Some industry leaders think the relationship between quality and productivity is exclusive, but Deming pointed out that productivity increases when quality improves because of less rework. When management is dedicated to producing a quality product or service, it empowers the workers to have pride in the quality of their work. As the labor process improves, the effects can be reduced mistakes, more uniform product output, and less waste of manpower, materials, or machine time. Benefits of this process also include lower costs, happier workers, and a better competitive position for the company [6] (Fig. 3-2).

Deming contends that support of top management for quality improvement is not enough. It takes total commitment and accountability that cannot be delegated to a lower level worker. Deming has become famous for his "Fourteen Points" that apply to any industry if the quality improvement process is to be successful[18]:

1. Create constancy of purpose for improvement of product and service.

    A company must develop a plan to become competitive and to stay in business through research, innovation, continuous improvement, and maintenance of improvement.

2. Adopt the new philosophy.

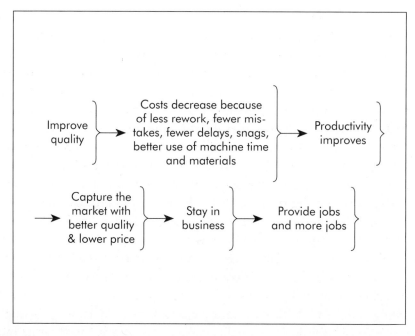

FIGURE 3-2
The Deming chain reaction. (From Deming WE: *Out of the crisis*, Cambridge, Mass, 1986, Massachusetts Institute of Technology.)

Americans must not tolerate poor service and workmanship. Americans must religiously reject mistakes and negativism.
3. Cease dependence on mass inspection.
American companies must eliminate need for inspection after the product is produced. When products are defective, the company pays for workers who made the products that must be either reworked or discarded. Quality comes from improving the production process, enlisting the workers involved when properly trained, rather than from inspection.
4. End the practice of awarding business on the basis of price tag.
Instead, industry leaders should depend on meaningful measures of quality, along with price. Seek the best quality supplier and build a long-term relationship to improve the quality.
5. Improve constantly and forever the system of production and service.

It is management's job to work continuously on the system to reduce waste and improve quality. Quality improvement is not a one-time effort or "program."

6. Institute training.

    Management must invest in training and not ask another worker who has never been trained to be the trainer. The worker cannot do the job because they have not been trained properly.

7. Institute leadership.

    The role of the supervisor is to lead not tell workers what to do. Leading means the supervisor helps the worker do better work and objectively evaluates who is need of individual assistance.

8. Drive out fear.

    Fear has a great economic loss. When people are afraid to ask questions or express their thoughts, the job may continue to be done wrong. To improve quality and productivity, the people must feel secure with management.

9. Break down barriers between staff areas.

    When departments, units, or areas have conflicting goals, competition may occur. This stops any teamwork toward finding opportunities for improvement.

10. Eliminate slogans, exhortations, and targets for the workforce.

    Quality is not a program with management-defined slogans. Let the people write their own slogans.

11. Eliminate numerical quotas.

    Quotas are only numbers and do not take quality or process methods into account. Quotas may be counterproductive because people will meet quotas to maintain a job although the company may suffer damage.

12. Remove barriers to pride of workmanship.

    People are eager to do a good job and want to do so. Management must remove barriers such as faulty equipment and defective materials, so the people can improve the quality of the product and process.

13. Institute a vigorous program of education and retraining.

    Management and workers must be educated and retrained in statistical techniques and teamwork for quality improvement to take place.

14. Take action to accomplish the transformation.

    It takes a dedicated team of top management with a defined action plan to lead the quality mission.

Both workers and management must understand the above "Fourteen Points," as well as the Seven Deadly Diseases and the Obstacles. Deming's Seven Deadly Diseases follow[18]:

1. Lack of constancy of purpose.

    A company without constancy of purpose has no strategic plan to stay in business. Employees and management are insecure without a plan.

2. Emphasis on short-term profits.

    When management concentrates on quarterly dividends alone, quality and productivity fall short.

3. Evaluation by performance, merit rating, or annual review of performance.

    These processes can destroy teamwork and increase rivalry among the people. They also can instill fear, leaving people despondent, and encourage management mobility.

4. Mobility of management.

    To be effective, management must be on the job long enough to understand the business and complete changes needed for improved productivity and quality. Job-hopping managers are detrimental to the company.

5. Running a company on visible figures alone.

    Often the unknown figures are the important ones such as the multiplier effect of a satisfied customer.

6. Excessive medical costs.

7. Excessive costs of warranty, fueled by lawyers who work for contingency fees.

Deming's "Obstacles" include neglect of long-range planning, expecting technology to solve problems, looking for examples to follow instead of seeking to develop the solutions, and excuses that impede quality improvement.[18]

Dr. J.M. Juran. Another famous leader in the field of quality is Dr. J.M. Juran. He was among the first to recognize that product quality does not happen by accident but rather is the result of careful planning. When a complacent America would not give Juran an ear, he took his concepts to

Japan in 1954. His teachings assisted the transition of Japanese interest movement from quality-control activities in technology to overall management concerns. Juran used statistical quality control as a management tool and established the concept of total-quality management as influenced by Dr. Armund V. Feigenbaum. Feigenbaum defined total quality control[10]:

> . . . an effective system for integrating the quality development, quality maintenance, and quality improvement efforts of various groups in an organization so as to enable production and service at the most economical levels which allow for full customer satisfaction.

As American industry experiences losses, ranging up to 40% of their yearly earnings because of poor quality control, Juran's principles are being looked to for assistance. He created the Juran Trilogy (Fig. 3-3), stating that there were three basic managerial processes to manage quality. They are quality planning, quality control, and quality improvement.[12] Many American companies such as AT&T, Caterpillar, DuPont, and IBM have embraced this trilogy.

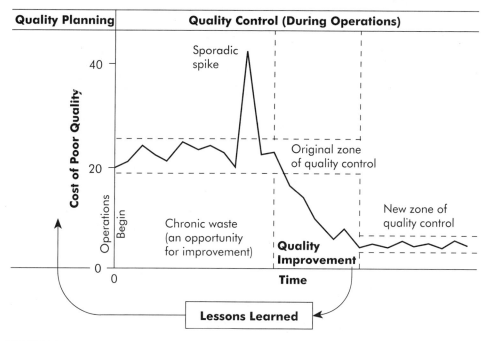

FIGURE 3-3
A, The Juran Trilogy diagram. (continued)

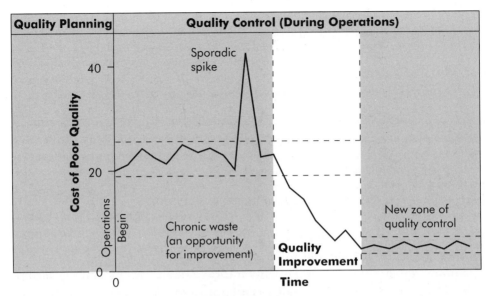

FIGURE 3-3 (continued).
B, Effect of quality improvement on operating results. **C,** The three universal processes of managing for quality. (From Juran JM: *Juran on leadership for quality,* New York, 1989, The Free Press.)

Juran provided a step-by-step guide for managers who want to implement quality planning. These include identification of customers and their needs, setting optimal quality goals, planning processes that can meet those goals under operating conditions, and producing continued results in market share, prices, and error-reduction rate in offices and factories.

Juran has developed eight success factors that characterize institutions that have improved quality and reduced quality-related costs[12]:

1. Senior managers personally led the quality process and served on a quality council as guides.
2. Managers applied quality improvement to businesses and traditional operational processes. These managers addressed internal and external customers.
3. The senior managers adopted mandated, annual quality improvement with a defined infrastructure that identified opportunities to improve and gave clear responsibility to do this.
4. The managers involved all those who affected the plan in the improvement process.
5. Managers used modern quality methodology instead of empiricism in quality planning.
6. Managers trained all members of the management hierarchy in quality planning, quality control, and quality improvement.
7. Managers trained the workforce to participate actively in quality improvement.
8. Senior managers included quality improvement in the strategic planning process.

Philip B. Crosby. Philip Crosby is considered another present-day expert in quality management. Crosby is chairman of a quality management consulting firm containing "Quality College." Before his success in the quality arena, he came up through the ranks of business as an "inspector, tester, assistant foreman, section chief, manager, director, and corporate vice president."[5]

Crosby is a consultant who believes that quality is free; what costs money are nonquality things, and all the time, manpower, and resources it takes to do things wrong the first time. Crosby says do it right the first time. He further contends that quality is a profit maker. It is this philosophy that led him to develop the quality management program at ITT.

Crosby assessed the need for corporate-wide emphasis on quality concerns. He then set about establishing a cultural revolution "that would last forever and become part of the corporate woodwork."[5] The program must be supported by four legs, namely[5]:
1. Management participation and attitude
2. Professional quality management
3. Original programs
4. Recognition

He called for management participation, not just support. He needed to dispel the popular myths about quality management: that quality meant goodness, error was inevitable, and people lacked concern for their work.[5]

Crosby defined quality as "conformance to requirements."[5] He taught management that it is always cheaper to do things right the first time. He also taught that the people in the units, or the workers, had the best ideas about why things were done wrong the first time. They were the ones subject to the designing, problems, and creations of someone in management without giving their own input into how the requirements could be met. This often resulted in error.

Crosby thought that quality managers were called to educate the top management about the importance of their job in quality management. They were not to perform the quality management function for the industry but rather to educate and guide workers and management in their jobs related to quality management. Crosby defines the quality management concept[5]:

> ... a systematic way of guaranteeing that organized activities happen the way they are planned. It is a management discipline concerned with preventing problems from occurring by creating the attitudes and controls that make prevention possible.

Other programs related to quality management that Crosby made famous are the Quality Management Maturity Grid, a grid that helps firms assess their progress in quality management; Zero Defects, a standard for management that conveys the "Do it Right the First Time" philosophy; Make Certain program, a defect prevention program for nonmanufacturing businesses; and the Quality Improvement Process. This last contribution consists of the following 14 steps that, according to Crosby, can turn any business around[5]:
1. Management commitment
2. Quality improvement team

3. Quality measurements
4. Cost of quality evaluation
5. Quality awareness
6. Corrective action
7. Establish an ad hoc committee for the Zero Defects program
8. Supervisor training
9. Zero defects day
10. Goal setting
11. Error cause removal
12. Recognition
13. Quality councils
14. Do it over again

Crosby puts great emphasis on the ways in which a business can "cost out" quality. This cost analysis would include all efforts in redoing tasks; all waste; warranties and handling this process; after service warranties, handling complaints; testing and inspection; and other costs of error.[5] He also suggests that terms such as "control" and "assurance" be replaced with just "quality" management.

Japanese vs. Western Quality Control

There are differences in the Japanese experience of quality control and that of United States and Western Europe. One such difference is in specialization. In the West, emphasis is placed on specialization and development of quality control as a profession. The person in charge of quality control answers any questions raised about the production process. Although this is one way of creating a highly skilled quality control specialist, the person's focus and vision are narrow. Contrary to this, in Japan more emphasis is placed on the ability of the worker to be a generalist. This does not necessarily produce the most highly skilled person in quality control but does make the worker more flexible in his or her abilities to serve the company.[11]

Another factor in Japanese success is the tendency toward a vertical society. In such a culture the workers have strong ties with the division chief. If a suggestion for quality control is made, the chief must suggest and implement the change. This is one reason why Deming's emphasis on CEO leadership in quality control was effective in Japan.[11]

The prevalence of labor unions has traditionally hindered implementing total quality control. In America functional labor unions control worker activity. If workers strike, the entire company often must shut down. In Japan the unions are enterprise-wide and allow workers to receive diverse training. Multiskilled activities are encouraged, and again, everyone can participate in quality control.[11]

Other factors to be considered in the success of Japanese quality control are management styles, elitism, and pay systems. In the West, scientific standards have been developed by the most talented and handed down for implementation by the worker. This attitude of little worker input into the work process is one reason absenteeism is so high in some Western companies. Workers often think they are machines and work for a livelihood. Work can be unsatisfying and boring. High turnover occurs. This is not a characteristic congruent with high-quality commitment to product and service delivery. In Japan the workers are often well educated and help set standards and work environment processes. Quality control is easier to accomplish.[11]

Along this same line of thought, the West may have an attitude of elitism in the area of education. Class consciousness can cause workers to resist the initial work experience because they think they are educated to higher work. In Japan so many workers are college graduates that this class consciousness has disappeared for the most part. One of Deming's "Seven Deadly Sins" is evaluation by performance, merit rating, and annual review of performance to increase pay rates. This assumes that people can be made more efficient through the incentive of money. Yet some say increased pay results in more absenteeism.

In Japan the work ethic involves understanding of human drives. The presence of joy, pleasure, and desire are considered for the worker. Monetary needs meet the very basic human desires. The more important desires are (1) satisfaction from a job well done, (2) happiness from cooperation with co-workers and proper recognition, and (3) the excitement of personal growth from developing abilities and achieving self-fulfillment.[11]

Quality Assessment in Industry

Quality assessment in industry has several steps. These must be in a form that can be understood by consumers and easy to implement by businesses. Some to consider are the following[11]:
1. Determine the assessment unit
2. Determine the measuring method
3. Determine the relative importance of quality characteristics

4. Arrive at a consensus on defects and flaws
5. Expose latent defectives
6. Observe quality statistically
7. "Quality of design" and "quality of conformance" (This is often called target quality. Quality of conformance implies conforming to the quality of design.)

"Quality assurance (assessment) is the very essence of quality control . . . to assure (assess) quality in a product so that a customer can buy it with confidence and use it for a long period of time with confidence and satisfaction."[11]

Quality Improvement Systems In Industry

The role of the worker must not be overlooked when quality management is initiated. In manufacturing, some industries have included workers effectively through the use of quality improvement teams. Education for workers on quality improvement is extremely important because the process is impossible without them, the actual producers. This involvement adds worker innovation and assumes worker ownership in the improvement process.

Quality circles and suggestion systems are another way to approach quality improvement. Several points must be emphasized as quality circles are implemented. First, participation cannot be mandated but must be voluntary. Each member must be willing to perform individual study to develop professionally. Likewise, the group must provide mutual development with increased cooperation with other teams. Finally, the eventual goal is total participation of all workers in the workplace quality circles.[11] Fig. 3-4 contrasts quality improvement teams and quality circles.

Quality Improvement: Six Steps to Implementation

To define further the steps in Deming's Plan-Do-Check-Action (PDCA) approach, the following may be helpful in implementing a quality improvement process[11]:
1. Determine goals and targets (these can be determined by policies)
2. Determine methods of reaching the goals (standardize the work)
3. Engage in education and training
4. Implement the work

Feature	QC Circles	Project Teams
Primary mission	To improve human relations	To improve quality
Secondary mission	To improve quality	To improve participation
Scope of project	Within a single department	Multidepartmental
Size of project	One of the useful many	One of the vital few
Membership	From a single department	From multiple departments
Basis of membership	Voluntary	Mandatory
Hierarchical status of members	Typically in the work force	Typically managerial or professional
Continuity	Circle remains intact, project after project	Team is ad hoc, disbands after project is completed

FIGURE 3-4
Contrast: QC circles and project teams. (From Juran JM: *Juran on leadership for quality,* New York, 1989, The Free Press.)

5. Check the effects of implementation (check causes, check through the efforts)
6. Take appropriate action

Several hindrances may be encountered in implementing a quality improvement process. These usually stem from processes designed by managers with no input from workers with poor attitudes. One major hurdle to overcome is the passivity of managers who avoid responsibility. Another is when people think they are doing things right and see no problems in the quality of present production or services. A third problem often encountered is egotists who think their own area is best, which impedes teamwork. The obstacle may be people who think their own way is best and think only of themselves or their own division. Again, these same people will volley for their own distinction.[11]

Teamwork is essential to continuous quality improvement. The human emotions of jealousy, despair, and envy are deterrents to quality improvement effectiveness. Another factor that sabotages quality improvement is people who are unaware of their immediate surroundings and/or insist on maintaining the past way of doing things. Any or all of these "people characteristics" can undermine quality improvement implementation.[11]

❖ QUALITY MANAGEMENT IN HEALTH CARE

In a similar way to industry, health care is trying to define "quality." Powerful organizations such as the Joint Commission for the Accreditation of Health Care Organizations (JCAHO), the American Medical Association (AMA), the American College of Surgeons (ACS), and the American Hospital Association (AHA) all search for the definition of quality with various approaches. The Health Care Financing Administration (HCFA) asks the same questions as it manages the federal health care budget.[3] This section looks at the evolution of many groups and influences in the search for quality management in health care.

History of Health Care Quality Review: JCAHO

As early as 1916 Dr. E.A. Codman expressed the need to review the medical practice of that time. He is known for spearheading the peer review process at Massachusetts General Hospital with systematic audits of the medical record.[13] The American College of Surgeons was formed in 1918 and required peer review of physicians, as well as other hospital departments. In 1951 the Joint Commission for the Accreditation of Hospitals (JCAH) took over this responsibility. The JCAH consisted of representatives from the American Hospital Association, American Dental Association, College of Practitioners, American Medical Association, College of Surgeons, and two consumers. This private, not-for-profit organization was charged with performing voluntary surveys with resulting accreditation and establishment of standards.

The Medicare regulations were initiated in 1965 with JCAH standards recognized as a benchmark of quality care. If a hospital was accredited by JCAH, it was automatically recognized as compliant with Medicare regulation. This cross-over recognition was known as "deemed status."

It was not until 1980 that JCAH actually put quality assurance into the standards. Before that, there was some reflection of quality assurance in medical staff standards, but 1980 changes gave force to addressing quality assurance in the hospital. This quality assurance focused on the "problem," with each department required to perform a set number of chart audits. This same year the utilization review standard was separated for individual consideration.

The JCAH changed direction in 1984. The focus was on the responsibility of the Board of Directors and department directors for routine data collection, trending, resolution, and follow-up. It was the following year, with the leadership change of Dr. Dennis O'Leary, that the JCAH took responsibility for standard revision and update to meet current quality needs in health care delivery.

In 1986 the Agenda for Change was initiated. Even the name of the agency was changed in 1987 to Joint Commission for the Accreditation of Health Care Organizations (JCAHO) to encompass all settings where health care is rendered. In 1988 the JCAHO finished the first part of the agenda with the completion of indicators for monitoring clinical performance in obstetrics and anesthesia.

Another major accomplishment was the final draft of the 12 key principles that characterize a quality health care organization[1]:

1. Mission
2. Culture
3. Strategic planning and resource programs
4. Organizational change
5. Role of the governing body, management, and clinical leadership
6. Leadership qualification, development, and assessment
7. Resources
8. Clinical competence of practitioners
9. Recruitment, development, evaluation, and retention policies and practices
10. Evaluation and improvement in patient care
11. Organizational integration and coordination
12. Continuity and comprehensiveness of care

These key principles will guide the JCAHO as it looks for clinical and organizational indicators of quality care and shows ways to improve that care. They also serve as the basis for rewriting accreditation standards. This task is not easy but will affect the provider's quality management processes and future accreditation status. In 1990, 17 test sites were named to begin pilot programs for input into indicators for this Agenda for Change.

The JCAHO currently accredits more than 5000 hospitals and more than 3000 other health care agencies. Their scope now covers the following[9]:
1. General and psychiatric hospitals
2. Nursing homes and other long-term care facilities
3. Psychiatric facilities such as substance abuse programs, community mental health, programs for the mentally retarded and developmentally disabled, and adult and adolescent psychiatric problems
4. Outpatient surgery programs, urgent care clinics, group practices, and community centers
5. Home care organizations
6. Managed care organizations

The governing board of JCAHO now consists of 24 members representing the American College of Surgeons, the American College of Physicians, the American Dental Association, the American Hospital Association, the American Medical Association, and three public members. The American Nurses' Association has asked for two seats. This is presently being considered.

Leaders in Quality Management in Health Care

Certain leaders have attempted to define quality in the service area of health care. Managers may struggle to decide exactly which leadership philosophy of quality improvement they want to follow. The most important point is to find a philosophy that works and stick to it. Variations will come as evolutions and changes occur over time. The following are several schools of thought.

Dr. Avedis Donabedian. The classic approach of quality assessment and improvement was assumed 20 years ago by Avedis Donabedian, M.D., M.P.H. Donabedian thought all systems included inputs, processes, and outputs but called them structure, process, and outcome. The inputs, or services, are combined with the processes, or care provided, to produce outcomes or outputs.[14] It is no wonder he has been called the dean of quality assessment.[3]

Donabedian further defines health care systems in terms of efficiency, or achieving a desired goal at minimum expense. Appropriateness is another component because this matches service with respect to a patient's specific health care need. Effectiveness, the last piece of this system, links the system to outcomes or outputs with the goal of improved or maintained health.[7]

In his last book Donabedian wrote an epilog that sums up his approach to quality management. He defined quality as "those attributes of the process of care that contribute to its desired outcomes."[8] He described the two components—technical competence and personal attention—as inseparable in defining the "quality."

The public and many professionals seem to fear that quality will be sacrificed with emphasis on cost. Donabedian states that by reducing redundant care the costs are naturally lowered. In fact he argues that eliminating unnecessary and harmful care improves the quality of care. As this is applied to current practice, one must address the ethical issue that underlies balancing costs with benefits in quality management.

Donabedian explores such topics as justification for surgery and resource use, or utilization management. Quality assessment is suggested to study occurrences of preventable adverse outcomes or achieving favorable outcomes. He also stressed data integrity and availability for use appropriately.

Dr. W. Edwards Deming. Dr. Deming again becomes an example of leadership when quality management in health care is discussed. He translated his famous "Fourteen Points" for quality management in health care.

Several health care systems have instituted Deming's process for quality and productivity management. One is the department of Quality-of-Care Management at the Harvard Community Health Plan, a large New England Health Maintenance Organization (HMO). Other excellent examples are the patient judgment systems developed by Hospital Corporation of America (HCA) to obtain patient feedback, only one part of its quality improvement process.[14]

Applying Industrial Models of Quality Management to Health Care Systems

Historically, health care providers assessed and monitored performance through quality assurance and determined if the performance conformed to standards. When there was a variance, quality improvement processes were implemented. This narrow approach may not be enough for quality management in today's environment. There are other consumers besides patients, such as third-party payors, who require quality.

Another limitation of a traditional quality approach is the static nature of standards that tends to settle on a given level of compliance and is rarely reassessed. What is the acceptable level of compliance and who sets this?

Often the focus in current health care quality management is on the physician. Modern quality management processes require system-wide changes that involve all professionals, departments, staff, and administration.

Another aspect of traditional quality assurance is the tendency to address specific aspects of physician performance, that is, technical expertise and interpersonal skills. There are other very important issues such as the physician's ability to mobilize facility resources and use these resources appropriately to provide quality care at reasonable costs in a timely fashion. An example is the doctor who forgets to sign verbal orders, resulting in wasted resources.[13]

Modern quality science uses statistical information and techniques to reach decisions. Industrial quality experts also emphasize that quality must be a continuous effort by all members of the organization to meet the needs and expectations of consumers. Management must lead this process with an empowered quality philosophy. This encourages open and honest discussion and leads the way to quality improvement.

Recognition, analysis, and minimization of variance is basic to industrial quality management. Because all aspects of health care display some variance, use of basic statistics is necessary. Use of control charts and other tools is essential. (Specific tools useful to statistical analysis in quality assessment and improvement are discussed in the appendix.) Some common crossovers for health care from industry include recognizing that processes are complex, that processes usually have unnecessary rework and wastes, and that personnel need training in simple analytical statistical techniques.[13]

National Demonstration Project On Quality Improvement in Health Care

The famous 1987 National Demonstration Project (NDP) was a successful effort to demonstrate the application of industrial quality management methods to health care delivery. Twenty-one U.S. health care organizations, including HMOs, hospitals, and group practices, were assigned a quality expert from major U.S. companies, consulting firms, and universities. The goal was to learn and use the quality consultant's expertise to improve the quality of some service at the health care organization. The project lasted only 8 months, but 17 health care facilities completed and reported a quality improvement project. Costs were covered by the The John A. Hartford Foundation; the time of the quality experts and organizational leaders was donated.

There were two limitations in the NDP. First, the quality improvement principle was used to work on medical organizational problems that resembled industrial problems. Few teams ventured into actual clinical areas. No team measured its success by improved patient health status, but the leaders believed this would be possible in organizations with mature quality management cultures. The second limitation was that the project was short in length and did not try to address a change in organizational culture. Berwick[2] states that for quality management to flourish, a transformation of culture must occur through adopting quality management.

Nonetheless, the results of the NDP are extraordinary and worthy of study by health care management. A list of participating organizations and quality advisors is provided in the appendix for further reference.[2]

❖ SUMMARY

There is a new emphasis on quality management in the industrial sector and for health care providers. There are more than 600 consultants teaching quality improvement with top salaries for lecturers reaching $10,000 a day.[15]

The *Wall Street Journal* carries news about health care quality and costs on a regular basis. A recent article claims three in every 1000 prescriptions are erroneous.[16] In 1988 the health expenditures in the United States rose to 10.44% of the gross national product with the result being stress and strain on the U.S. citizens to pay for quality health care.[17]

Businesses are approaching the government for answers as the costs and demand for quality rises. Hewlett Packard officials recently stated that the center of attention is really quality issues. Providers have a choice to make care decisions on measures of quality or strictly on measures of cost.[4] A recent letter to a hospital president stated that the Prudential Insurance Company of America is committed to be a responsible a participant in the health care delivery system. They want to offer their clients high quality care at competitive prices. Their proposal was the Institutes of Quality network composed of physicians and facilities who have superior patient care outcomes. The hospital president was invited to provide information requested for use in this network.

As Americans face the 1990s, quality management is sure to be a major focus of health care, as well as business. There are several models that have been proposed, and many more will evolve. A major emphasis is on the responsibility of management to direct the quality philosophy. There is no better time than now for nursing administrators to demonstrate excellence in quality management.

REFERENCES
1. *Agenda for Change Update*, 2(1), June 1988, JCAHO.
2. Berwick DM, Godfrey AB, Roessner, J: *Curing health care: new strategies for quality improvement*, San Francisco, 1990, Jossey-Bass.
3. Buckland, AE: In search of . . . quality, *J Am Med Rec Assoc* 60(3): 1989.
4. Business leaders bring their clout to Washington, *Hospitals*, April 20, 1990.
5. Crosby PB: *Quality is free*, New York, 1979, American Library.
6. Deming WE: *Quality, productivity, and competitive position*. Cambridge, Mass, 1982, Massachusetts Institute of Technology Center for Advanced Engineering Study.
7. Donabedian A: *Aspects of medical care administration: specifying requirements for health care*, Cambridge, Mass, 1973, Harvard University Press for the Commonwealth Fund.
8. Donabedian A: *Explorations in Quality Assessments and Monitoring, vol 3*. Ann Arbor, 1984, Health Administration Press.
9. *Facts About the Joint Commission*, Chicago, 1990, JCAHO.
10. Feigenbaum AV: *Total quality control*, New York, 1983, McGraw-Hill.
11. Ishikawa K: *What is total quality control? The Japanese way*, New Jersey, 1985, Prentice-Hall.
12. Juran JM: *Juran on planning for quality*, New York, 1988, Free Press.
13. Laffel G, Blumenthal D: The case for using industrial quality management science in health care organizations, *JAMA* 262(20): 1989.
14. Lanning J, O'Conner S: The health care quality quagmire: some signposts, *Hospital & Health Services Administration*, 35(1):41, 1990.
15. Special Report: The U.S. and quality: a new culture, *Industry Week*, April 17, 1989.
16. *Wall Street Journal*, May 2, 1990.
17. *Wall Street Journal*, May 2, 1990.
18. Walton M: *The Deming management method*, New York, 1986, Putnam.

CHAPTER 4

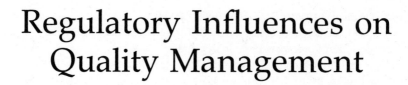

Regulatory Influences on Quality Management

❖ INTRODUCTION

INNUMERABLE laws and regulations affect all aspects of health care delivery, quality, types of services provided, and reimbursement for services. Many third-party payors are joining the government's efforts in the quest for high-quality care at a reasonable price. Federal agencies and many private insurance companies specify what types of care can be provided and in what setting. The provision of quality, cost-effective care entails timely, efficient use of all technology, medicines, therapies, services, and available resources. Knowledge of historical and regulatory influences on health care delivery and reimbursement is essential to understanding the current activities and future trends. Tailoring care to meet the needs of the individual is at the forefront of promoting quality and containing cost. This chapter will include a historical review of the origins of health care insurance and how technology and medical advances have affected cost.

❖ THE HISTORY OF HEALTH INSURANCE

The beginnings of health insurance can be traced to the seventeenth and eighteenth centuries in London. Workers could pay a specified amount to ensure that their family would receive health care if they became ill. The practice worked well until 1831, when a cholera epidemic occurred, and there were insufficient funds to cover the needs of so many.

In the United States before the Depression of the 1930s health care was very simplistic. There were no advanced technologies or medicines. Many of the prevalent medical practices were simple remedies. Cost for this primitive care was nominal. Services of a physician were based on a fee-for-service concept, meaning an ill person saw the physician and paid at the end of the visit. The average person could most likely afford any health care services needed. Hospitals were supported mostly by charitable donations. If a person could not pay his or her expenses, the donations supposedly paid for his or her care, although charity care was not the high quality of care received by a patient who could afford to pay. During the Depression, the average American could not afford the cost of health care. Because of this and the immense drop in charitable donations, many hospitals faced closure. Insurance protection was nonexistent; nor was there any federal, state, or local funding available to defray costs. There were a few forms of disability insurance where the employer paid a portion of an employee's salary to the family when an employee was ill, but generally there was no illness coverage.

The development of antibiotics and the technologic advances in the 1940s had both positive and negative effects on health care delivery. Although these advances had the ability to improve health for many, the cost was prohibitive for many average Americans. Based on increasing cost and the inability of people to pay, some envisioned a prepaid payment system that would relieve the burden to the individual in the event of an illness. The creation of health insurance would benefit the individual and would assure that hospital and physician expenses were paid.

The first known insurance in the United States was developed in 1927 by a physician, Michael Shadid, in Elk City, Oklahoma. The people in the community bought shares from the physician to build a hospital in their community. In turn, the shareholders would receive any needed medical care. In 1929 a prepaid program for teachers was established in Dallas, a creation of Justin Ford Kimball at the Baylor University Hospital. That same year in Los Angeles a prepaid coverage system was created for municipal employees, funded by Dr. Donald Ross and Clifford Loos. The Kaiser-Permanente network emerged as a result of a relationship between Henry Kaiser and Dr. Sidney Garfield. Ship workers could enroll in a prepaid health insurance program. The cost for the program was underwritten by an insurance company owned by Kaiser.

Prepaid health programs were resisted by legislators and physicians, who believed that prepaid health programs stifled free enterprise and affected quality of care. In spite of the resistance the American Hospital Association (AHA) recognized the appeal of prepaid programs and developed national standards governing these programs in 1933, based on the Baylor Hospital plan. Physicians, legislators, and hospitals collaborated to create the first Blue Cross plan, which was introduced in 1939, and in 1941 a plan was introduced that covered physicians.

❖ GOVERNMENT SUPPORT FOR HEALTH CARE EXPANSION

When the technologic advances occurred, there was an era of health care expansion from the 1940s through the 1960s. Much of this expansion was promoted and funded by the federal government. The Hospital Survey and Construction Act of 1946, known as the Hill-Burton Act, marked the beginning of extensive federal subsidization for the creation of health resources to facilitate access to care. Many hospitals were built, particularly in rural areas.

Continued medical research and technologic progress were made possible by the National Institutes of Health. Federal funding and support promoted the medical education and education for other health care personnel. The policies of this period were geared to increased access to quality health care.

Private insurance growth, dating to the 1940s, the Hill-Burton Act, which stimulated hospital building, and the creation of Medicare and Medicaid were all aimed at access to quality health care as the right of each individual (see Box on p. 47).

❖ MEDICARE

Medicare and Medicaid, introduced in 1965, were designed to decrease the financial barriers for health care for the elderly, the poor, and any persons 65 or older who were entitled to Social Security or railroad retirement (see Box on p. 47). In 1963 a Social Security survey indicated that approximately one half of the retirees had no private health insurance. It was common for a person to lose his or her employer-sponsored health insurance. Comprehensive policies for the elderly were essentially nonexistent, and insurance companies feared insuring the elderly. The policies that were available were generally inadequate or offered limited coverage. In 1973 legislation was passed to extend Medicare coverage to the permanently and

> ### *Government Support for Health Care Expansion*
>
> 1946—Hill-Burton Act
> 1965—Medicare/Medicaid legislation
> 1973—Expanded Medicare to cover permanently or totally disabled, end-stage renal disease

totally disabled. Coverage also was extended to patients with end-stage renal disease (see Box above). Hospital utilization increased and was directly attributable to the Medicare population. Part A covered inpatient care and was funded totally by federal funds. Part B covered outpatient services and was voluntary. It was partially funded by the government and partially by payments from the individual. Inflation, expanding technology, and Medicare enrollment causing increased demand affected the increase of Medicare outlay by federal government.

Medicaid was a companion piece to Medicare. It was enacted to provide federal assistance to the states to aid in providing health care to the poor. Although this program was a joint attempt of both the federal and state governments, the administrative responsibility for operation was given to the individual states. Homemaker services were social services that were covered services of Medicaid, but because of cost concerns, most states elected not to provide these. In some cases people were eligible for both Medicare and Medicaid and were termed dually eligible. This included a group of frail, elderly, poor persons. Studies have shown this group to have higher utilization of resources and services.

❖ 1970s—THE COST CONTAINMENT ERA

The federal government realized in the early 1970s that it could not afford unlimited coverage for unlimited numbers of enrollees in Medicare. Some of the key cost containment policies addressed utilization review, rate control, and control of capital expenditures. A witness to the changing thought was the 1972 amendments to the Social Security Act, creating the Professional Standards Review Organization (PSRO). Physicians were given the responsibility to review Medicare patients, to control health care utilization and ultimately the cost. The Economic Stabilization Program created during the Nixon Administration was an attempt to control hospital rates and was in effect from 1971 to 1974. The major objective of rate control was cost containment; although there was a federal program to control rates, the burden for rate control fell on the individual states. Congress passed the National Health Planning and Resources Development Act in 1974. This legislation authorized and established a national certificate-of-need (CON) program intended to control capital expansion in the health sector. Its objectives were the following:

1. Improving the health of residents of a health service area
2. Increasing accessibility (including overcoming geographic, architectural, and transportation barriers), acceptability, continuity, and quality of health services
3. Restraining increases in cost of providing services
4. Preventing unnecessary duplication of health services

❖ THE 1980s POLICY SHIFT

By the early 1980s, the federal government realized it could not meet its health care financial objectives by mere regulation. Legislation therefore was created that exhibited a blend of regulatory and market strategies. The passage of the Omnibus Budget Reconciliation Act of 1981 and the Tax Equity and Fiscal Responsibility Act (TEFRA) of 1982 was a combination of both. These laws placed regulatory limits on ancillary services provided by hospitals, but the law permitted Health Maintenance Organizations (HMOs) to offer competitive medical plans and participate in care designed to foster competition. The 1982 TEFRA Act replaced per diem cost limits with operating cost-per-case limits and mandated the development of a prospective pricing system. Also in 1982 the Peer Review Improvement Act repealed the PSRO program, replacing it with the Peer Review Organization (PRO). In 1983 the Social Security Amendment established the role of the PRO to "review physicians and other health care providers in multiple settings." The Health Care Financing Administration (HCFA) issued requests from those organizations wishing to become PROs.

The prospective pricing based on diagnostic related groups (DRGs) came with the passage of the Social Security Amendment of 1983. This legislation was again an attempt to control utilization and ultimately cost. The National Health Planning and Resource Development Act was repealed in 1986, which was a repeal of the certificate-of-need (CON) requirement. Health

CHAPTER 4   REGULATORY INFLUENCES ON QUALITY MANAGEMENT   **49**

Cost Containment Era/Federal Government

1971-74	Economic Stabilization Program
1972	PSRO Creation
1974	National Health Planning and Resources Development Act
1982	TEFRA
1982	Peer Review Improvement Act
1983	Prospective pricing based on DRGs

---

care services were becoming more competitive and the adoption of legislation was reinforcing the trend (see Box above).

❖ CHAMPUS

CHAMPUS insurance describes an insurance plan created for Civilian Health and Medical Programs of the Uniformed Services. In 1984 the Department of Defense Authorization Act gave CHAMPUS authority to reimburse institutional providers based on Diagnostic Related Groups (DRGs). The Consolidated Omnibus Budget Reconciliation Act of 1985 took effect January 1, 1987. Medicare participating hospitals were required to accept patients from CHAMPUS. In October 1987 CHAMPUS implemented a DRG-based payment system modeled after the Medicare prospective pricing system. The Peer Review Organization reviews CHAMPUS just as it reviews Medicare, utilizing the same generic screening tools.

The Joint Commission on Accreditation (JCOA) was established in 1948 as a voluntary, independent accrediting organization. The original Joint Commission enlisted members from the American Hospital Association, the American Medical Association, the American Dental Association, the American College of Practitioners and Surgeons, and two consumers. Hospital accreditation standards were first published by the Joint Commission in 1953.

In 1965, the same year Medicaid and Medicare were established, HCFA gave the Joint Commission what was called deemed status. The HCFA gave the Joint Commission standards as the benchmark of quality and as meeting most of Medicare standards. The JCAHO has continually revised and amended the standards to reflect changes in approach to health care and technology. In 1970 the Joint Commission shifted the standards from reviewing minimum requirements to what was considered an optimum level. It utilized retrospective medical care audits to review patient care. By 1975 the JCAHO standards required medical and professional groups to evaluate the quality of patient care by establishing explicit, measurable criteria. In 1980 the first Joint Commission quality assessment standard was introduced. A revision of that standard followed in 1985. The focus became routine data collection and periodic assessment. Great emphasis was placed on the responsibilities of the board members of an institution. Systemwide, ongoing evaluation and monitoring was emphasized. In 1986 the Agenda for Change initiatives began. Once again the Joint Commission was redefining and refocusing emphasis[6]:

> As the Joint Commission enters the 1990s, we begin an era of accreditation and service to health care organizations, their professional staffs, and the American public. Much of the groundwork for the new era was laid in 1986 with the introduction of the Agenda for Change initiatives. Through these innovative changes, the Joint Commission once again set out to take the lead in improving the quality of health care in the United States. The Joint Commission's many decades of experience as a standard setter and evaluator of health care quality led to the identification of two critical interdependent factors in the provision of quality health care—careful ongoing attention to the process and outcomes of care and emphasis on continuous improvement in patient care services. These two thrusts form the bedrock of the Agenda for Change objectives. Increased attention to the process and outcome of services and emphasis on continuous improvement are interdependent factors in providing quality service, whether in patient care or in the Joint Commission accreditation and educational activities.

Into the 1990s the JCAHO will continue to focus on processes and outcomes as it moves toward continuous quality improvement.

❖ PEER REVIEW ORGANIZATION

The Peer Review Organization (PRO) was created in 1982 by the Peer Review Improvement Act. In 1983 in a Social Security amendment, the role of the PRO was expanded to include review of other health care practitioners in addition to physicians. This review included review in institutional and noninstitutional settings. HCFA issued a request in 1984, soliciting those who wanted to become Peer Review Organizations.

In 1986 HCFA required the PRO to use generic screens on all chart reviews. The use of generic screens was an attempt to standardize criteria used for review and to measure all health care services using the same basic criteria. In 1986 amendments to the Omnibus Budget Reconciliation Act further defined the realm of PRO by addressing services provided in Ambulatory Surgery Centers, further defining DRGs and requiring that all patients receive discharge planning.

The Health Care Quality Improvement Act created a centralized data bank. This data bank serves as a source of information regarding health care providers. This data source gives information regarding informal proceedings against a health care provider for what would be considered negligent or imprudent services rendered. From the creation of the PRO until the present, legislative changes have promoted the expansion of the role of the PRO. This expansion includes redefining and refining the review process, as well as expansion into all facets of health care.

❖ MANAGED CARE

Managed care is a term used to describe several types of health care coverage. Managed care is an approach to health care in which the objective is to arrange care that is comprehensive and coordinated, at the most appropriate level, and at the most cost-effective price. Managed care encompasses several types of systems, which include Health Maintenance Organizations (HMOs), Individual Practice Associations (IPAs), and Preferred Provider Organizations (PPOs). Characteristics of these plans are prepayment, comprehensive coverage, and preventive care.

Health Maintenance Organizations

A Health Maintenance Organization (HMO) is a prepaid health care program in which services are provided by a group to a group[8]:

> According to the U.S. Department of Health and Human Services, which is responsible for the provisions of the HMO Act of 1973, it is a managed health care plan that provides or arranges for the delivery of comprehensive, coordinated medical services to voluntarily enrolled members on a prepaid basis. The key phrase that separates HMOs from other forms of health care delivery coverage is managed care. It means that someone is overseeing the cost and quality of our care, as well as our use of that care.

Throughout the 1940s and 1950s, labor and trade unions argued for full coverage at a lower cost to the consumer/patient with no compromise in quality. The Teamsters in St. Louis, the United Mine Workers in Appalachia, and the United Auto Workers in Detroit established prepaid group practices for their members. The Kaiser-Permanente HMO was the forerunner of today's HMOs. The HMO concept grew to such proportion that in 1973 the Health Maintenance Organization Act was passed. This legislation standardized the development of HMOs and provided financial support for established HMOs. Health Maintenance Organizations that are public or private come under this legislation. This enactment specified the types of services to be provided and the manner in which the HMO was to be organized. Industries that have HMOs were required to offer employees the option of health insurance as opposed to an HMO. The legislation further required that the governing board of an HMO consists of no less than one third of its customers. From 1973 until the present there has been continual growth of the HMO managed care concept. In 1979 an amendment to the original 1973 legislation attempted to address HMOs in relation to alternative delivery such as skilled care units and home health.

The HMO concept arose from a need to provide quality health care and control costs, providing care to those on fixed incomes and in underserved areas where quality providers were unavailable. The emphasis in an HMO is ambulatory care, prevention, and efficiency. The healthier the membership, the fewer dollars spent.

Independent Practice Associations

The Independent Practice Association (IPA) is a fast-growing variation of the HMO concept. It is a prepaid health care plan offered by a group of physicians in private practice to a group of members. The clients can see any physician who is a member of the IPA. In an IPA, members are not billed for physician services, but physicians are paid for every visit. Their referral system is essential to the viability of the IPA. The primary care physician serves as the gatekeeper by referring patients to other physicians in the IPA.

Preferred Provider Organizations

Preferred Provider Organizations (PPOs) are another form of managed care. The most distinct characteristic of a PPO is that it is an open-use system based on a negotiated fee schedule. Patients have a choice of use of a PPO physician or not. If they choose a non-PPO physician, the PPO pays a smaller portion of the cost of the visit, and the physician sets his or her own fee. The nonmember physician will bill a patient for the difference in what the PPO pays and the fee for his or her service.

❖ HOW UTILIZATION MANAGEMENT IS AFFECTED

Technologic advances and increased cost for health care have been the driving force in the need for utilization management. As programs developed to help defray cost to the individual consumer, there has been a need to control outlay by insurance companies and federal-and state-funded health delivery programs. In addition, the creation of other health insurance concepts such as HMOs has forced the HMO and the providers to look at utilization of services and appropriateness as part of quality care. Utilization management is inherent in the health delivery systems and those responsible for the payment for services. Effective utilization management can ensure viability of a health care provider, viability of the insurance carrier, and quality appropriate care to the individual.

❖ SUMMARY

The Depression and technologic advances influenced the creation of insurance and the development of managed care programs. The Kaiser-Permanente program was the forerunner of today's Health Maintenance Organizations. Many other programs of insurance coverage emerged despite the fears of physicians and legislators that the prepaid programs stifled free enterprise and negatively affected quality.

In 1933 the American Hospital Association developed national standards for prepaid programs. Physicians and legislators collaborated to create the Blue Cross plan in 1939. A third-party payment system was devised in an effort to control cost and monitor quality.

Government support for health was evident by the passage of the Hospital Survey and Construction Act of 1946, better known as the Hill-Burton Act, for hospital building programs and funds for medical and health care personnel education. In 1965 an amendment to the 1935 Social Security Act created Medicare and Medicaid. These programs increased access of health care to the poor and elderly. In 1973 legislation was passed extending coverage to the disabled and to those with end-stage renal disease. This caused a major increase in the enrollment numbers.

The 1970s became the era of cost-containment. The government realized it could not afford unlimited coverage for unlimited numbers of enrollees. One of the first steps in utilization control and ultimately cost containment was the 1972 amendment to the Social Security Act that created the Peer Review Standards Organization (PRSO). Physicians were given the responsibility for this review. The Economic Stabilization Program under the Nixon Administration and the National Health Planning and Resources Development Act were attempts to control hospital rates and control capital expansion by developing a "certificate of need" (CON) program. The government's objectives were to improve health for all, to increase accessibility, to restrain cost, and to prevent unnecessary duplication of health services.

Prospective pricing for care was a result of the 1982 Tax Equity and Fiscal Responsibility Act. The Peer Review Standards Organization was replaced by the Peer Review Organization (PRO). The National Health Planning and Resources Act, which created CON laws, was repealed in 1986, thus showing a shift toward competition. Legislation attempted to control cost yet stimulate a competitive market for health care providers.

The Joint Commission on Accreditation was established in 1948 as a voluntary, independent accrediting organization. In 1965 the Health Care Financing Administration gave the Joint Commission deemed status, thus recognizing that organization as the benchmark for quality and the closest to approximating Medicare standards. In 1970 the Joint Commission shifted its standards from review of minimum requirements to optimum level of care. In 1975 JCAH required review of care by professionals based on the establishment of explicit, measurable criteria. The Joint Commission established a quality assessment standard in 1980 with a revision in 1985. From 1986 until the present the Agenda for Change initiatives are the focus. The bedrock for the Agenda for Change is increased attention to process and outcome of services.

The Peer Review Organization was established in 1982 with expansion of review beyond physicians in 1983. Many of the organizations that responded to the call to be PROs were former PSRO groups. In 1986 HCFA required the PRO to use generic screening and redefining, and the development of an expanded role is seen emerging.

Managed care is a concept that encompasses several types of systems. Characteristics of managed care plans include prepayment, comprehensive coverage, and preventive care. The HMO Act of 1973 was designed to regulate HMO development. Independent Practice Associations (IPAs) are a variation of the HMO concept where prepaid health care is provided to members by a group of physicians in private practice. Preferred Provider Organizations (PPOs) are another form of managed care, which is an open-use system based on a negotiated fee schedule.

Health care costs and quality concerns have been the driving force in the need for utilization management programs. Effective utilization management can benefit the patient by assuring quality health care that is appropriate. Utilization management also can help to control costs, ensuring the viability of insurance, the carrier, as well as the institutional provider. The creation of DRGs and prospective pricing has drawn attention to the need for an effective utilization management program to control cost, monitor quality, and ensure overall appropriateness and continued availability of services.

REFERENCES

1. Clark MJD: *Community nursing: health care for today and tomorrow,* Reston, Va, 1984, Reston Publishing.
2. Coile, RC: Managed care: 10 leading trends for the 1990s, II. *Aspens Advisor* 5(1):1-8, 1990.
3. Greaney FJ: Opportunities for nurses in utilization review, *Nursing economics,* 41(5): 1986.
4. Grimaldi PL: National medicare PPS rates are here, *Nursing management,* 18(11):22-24, 1987.
5. Jewler D: Cutting through the red tape, *Diabetes Forecast,* pp. 58-59, 61-62, July 1988.
6. Joint Commission on Accreditation of Healthcare Organizations: Agenda for Change, Chicago, Joint Commission, 1990.
7. Kilbee P: *The national association of quality assurance professionals, quality assurance and risk management:* a study guide and primer, 1989, National Association for Quality Assurance Professionals.
8. Longest, BB, Jr: American health policy in the year 2000, Hospital and health services administration 33(4): 419-434, 1988.
9. McGovern KJ, Newborn VB: Long-term care facility DRG impact, *Gerontol Nurse* 14(9):17-20, 38-39 1988.
10. *Mid South Foundation for Medical Care Manual,* Tennessee Peer Review Organization, 1990.
11. Miller DB, Barry JT: *Nursing home organization and operation,* 1979.

CHAPTER 5

Quality Assurance/ Quality Improvement

Sandra S. Bassett

❖ DEFINITION

QUALITY patient care has become an important factor in the health care arena. For years quality has been assumed; now, many different types of customers are requesting evidence of quality. Before one measures quality, one must define it. The definition varies according to the user or consumer. Donabedian, a leader in medical quality assurance, initially defined quality as, "that kind of care which is expected to maximize an inclusive measure of patient welfare, after one has taken account of the balance of expected gains and losses that attend the process of care in all its parts."[4] In recent years experts have applied the industrial definition to health care with a focus on continuous efforts by all employees to meet the needs of the customer. The Joint Commission on Accreditation of Healthcare Organizations (JCAHO) embraces the following definition of quality, "the degree to which patient care services increase the probability of desired patient outcomes and reduce the probability of undesired outcomes, given the current state of knowledge."[1] As W. Edwards Deming concludes, quality has meaning only in terms of the customer.

❖ HISTORY

To understand the relationship of quality assurance (QA) to quality improvement (QI), one must have an understanding of the underlying history.

Quality assurance actually began in the early 1900s as part of the minimum standards of the American College of Surgeons (ACS). Although the standards were not called QA, the organization did require regular review and evaluation of the quality of care provided to hospitalized patients. Later, JCAHO assumed the responsibilities of the ACS and began to develop standards that paralleled the minimum standards. In the beginning the review processes were informal, subjective in nature, and based on the reviewer's knowledge and experience. During this time researchers were developing methods that focused on objectivity and structure. Although the mechanisms were contrasting, both utilized systematic review procedures and developed objective, valid criteria for the review process. With this in place JCAHO advocated medical audit methodology in the early 1970s that resulted in retrospective outcome-oriented audits.[9] By 1980 JCAHO had written its first standard on quality assurance. During the next several years the requirements ranged from medical audits to problem-focused studies to ongoing monitoring and evaluation processes. Health care facilities clearly moved away from "problem of the month" or crisis management based on individual occurrences.

During the mid-1980s the Joint Commission developed the Agenda for Change, a major developmental project intended to create an outcome-oriented monitoring and evaluation process that could help organizations improve the quality of care they provide.[5] Task forces developed outcome indicators in the areas of obstetrics, anesthesia, oncology, cardiovascular, trauma, medication usage, infection control, and home care. Other areas were targeted for future development of indicators. Facilities of different sizes and different geographic locations were selected by JCAHO to test the indicators' usefulness and data availability. After extensive field review, accredited organizations will be required to collect and submit the data to JCAHO. The facilities' response to the data will be used in the accreditation process. In addition to the development of outcome indicators the Agenda for Change focuses on continuous improvement. Health care organizations that are accreditated by JCAHO will be challenged to address improvement in quality of care with creative and innovative approaches.

❖ QUALITY ASSURANCE VERSUS QUALITY IMPROVEMENT

Quality assurance and quality improvement are not synonymous but complement and enhance each other (see Table 5–1). According to a report

Table 5–1 Quality Assurance Versus Quality Improvement

Quality Assurance	Quality Improvement
QA	QI
Inspection oriented (detection)	Planning oriented (prevention)
Reactive	Proactive
Correction of special clauses (individual, machine)	Correction of common causes (system)
Responsibility of few	Responsibility of all
Narrow focus	Cross-functional
Leadership may not be vested	Leadership actively leading
Problem solving by authority	Problem solving by employees at all levels

to the American Hospital Association, continuous quality improvement is nearly always built on the foundation of good ongoing quality review.[6] Unlike QA, QI is a total process that requires a change in management philosophy and overall culture. Quality improvement must permeate the entire organization beginning with top administration. It encourages creativity, intra- and interdepartmental communication, and cooperation at all times. Quality assurance focuses primarily on clinical aspects of care and practitioner performance. Quality improvement focuses on processes of service and/or care, as well as the customer's perceptions of care. Quality improvement processes were adapted from industrial quality control theories established mainly by W. Edwards Deming, J.M. Juran, and Walter Shewhart. Japanese companies began using the QI concept in the 1950s.

As organizations began embarking on the quality improvement process, many were skeptical whether the model could be applied to the health care setting with the same success as Japanese companies. To explore this question, the National Demonstration Project on Quality Improvement in Health Care was initiated. Quality experts from the industrial side were paired with teams from 21 health care organizations. The results from the project are reported by Donald Berwick in his book *Curing Health Care*. The organizations successfully applied simple industrial tools to demonstrate processes of care and to reveal causes of variation. With a clear, visual definition of the problem or opportunity, the teams were able to address the issues, which resulted in improvements. The overall conclusion was that quality improvement tools can be applied to the health care setting.[2]

❖ QUALITY ASSESSMENT/IMPROVEMENT PROCESS IN NURSING ROLES AND RESPONSIBILITIES

Although the governing body is ultimately responsible for the care and services rendered by the organization, each individual is responsible for improving care. The responsibility for nursing quality improvement is delegated down through the facility's management structure to the nursing administrator. The commitment and degree of involvement by the staff nurse is directly related to participation and ownership of the process. The program must be tailored to the facility, based on size, available resources, patient/customer expectation, availability of staff, and time allocation. Education relative to QI falls to nurse educators and administrators. Because there are limited resources for education, managers responsible for coordinating the program must be motivated to learn on their own. Many universities have developed curricula regarding quality improvement. Once the initial education is complete for the staff, the next challenge for nurse administrators is to sustain an appropriate level of motivation and commitment to ensure an effective quality assessment/quality improvement process.

❖ PROCESS DEVELOPMENT

Because regulatory or accreditation agencies do not mandate the components or structure of a quality improvement process, the development of the process is at the discretion of the nurse administrator. Under the old school of thought, many centralized processes were controlled and implemented by one individual, with little staff involvement. However, the most successful structure is decentralized or unit-based, which promotes participation and ownership. The department of nursing services' plan incorporates each unit's plan. The quality assessment plan should be workable, simplistic, and understandable. The key factor is to determine if the process accomplishes what the plan purports to do; that is, does it work for nursing services?

A committee structure is often utilized at the unit level with the chairman reporting to the overall nursing QI committee structure. In turn, the chairman would report to the facility-wide committee. Many hospitals have found that the QI program is just as successful without a committee but functions well with a quality improvement coordinator. In addition to the coordination activities the staff person would provide education relating to QI, ensure appropriate communication of activities, facilitate team activities, and be a resource to all staff.

❖ JCAHO'S 10-STEP MONITORING AND EVALUATION PROCESS

According to JCAHO the concept of continuous quality improvement incorporates the strengths of quality assurance while broadening its scope. The current JCAHO's 10-step model[10] can be used as a basis for establishing an effective quality assessment and improvement process. The process, which focuses on monitoring, evaluating, and problem solving, is designed to assist an organization to effectively use its resources to manage the quality of care it provides. Under this model, the activities are ongoing, planned, systematic, and comprehensive. They are designed so that data collection, evaluation, and problem-solving activities are adequate to identify opportunities or problems. Expansions of this model include (1) the role of leadership in the process, (2) extension of activities into all areas, not just clinical, (3) identification of customer and supplier relationships, and (4) focusing on process of care and services rather than on individual performance or outliers (see box below: see Chapter 5 Appendix for further information).

Step 1: Assign Responsibility

As stated previously the governing body has the ultimate responsibility of patient/client care. The organizational leaders are responsible for setting the stage by fostering an atmosphere that focuses on continuously improving care. According to JCAHO the organizational leaders should include at least the leaders of the governing body, medical staff, managerial staff, and the nurse executive. The nurse executive oversees and sets the priority assessment and improvement activities within all areas where nursing care is provided.

JCAHO'S 10-Step Monitoring and Evaluation Process

1. Assign responsibility
2. Delineate scope of care
3. Identify important aspects of care
4. Identify indicators
5. Establish thresholds for evaluation
6. Collect and organize data
7. Evaluate care
8. Take action to improve care
9. Assess actions and document improvement
10. Communicate information

Step 2: Delineate Scope of Care

The scope of care can be delineated using one of two methods—identifying activities and identifying key functions. When using the identification of activities method, the who, what, when, and where relative to the services or care provided determine the scope of care. The following should be included: types of patients served; conditions or diagnosis treated; services, treatments, or activities performed; types of practitioners providing the care; sites of service; and times of service delivery. This provides a comprehensive inventory of the facility or department.

The second method is to identify the organization's key governance, managerial, clinical, and support functions. The process involves all departments and services. Key functions relate to those that have the greatest effect or impact on the quality of care. JCAHO will stress using this method more in the future.

Regardless of the method used in delineating the scope of care, the focus of quality improvement will be understanding the processes involved and improving related activities. The priority in which the activities are addressed is dependent on the customer and supplier relationship. Each subsequent step is based on the scope of care.

Step 3: Identify Important Aspects of Care

Aspects of care are determined by their degree of importance. Because of limited resources, review must focus on those areas that have the greatest impact on patient care. According to the JCAHO model, priority of review should be assigned to aspects of care in which one or more of the following is true:

1. High volume (HV): Occurs frequently or affects large numbers of patients.
2. High risk (HR): Has demonstrated patients at risk for serious consequences or are deprived of substantial benefit if the care is not provided correctly, in a timely manner, or for the proper identification.
3. Problem-prone (PP): Has tended to produce problems for staff or patient and/or significant other.

As changes in reimbursement and shift of care from acute care setting continue to be major issues, cost of the product or service could be another consideration.

Aspects of care can relate to key functions, procedures, treatments, activities, or processes of care. As the important aspects of care are identified, assign one or more of the categories to them. This will clearly demonstrate the reason for selection for review and assist with priority placement. Even though the department of nursing services may not be able to monitor and evaluate each area during the year, it is important to identify all aspects of care based on the department's scope.

Step 4: Identify Indicators

For each important aspect of care, at least one indicator should be identified. An indicator is a quantitative measure that can be used as a guide to monitor and evaluate the quality of patient care. An indicator is not a direct measure of quality but a screen or flag that may indicate a need for further investigation.[8] The indicator should be well defined, comprehensive, relevant, efficient, and clinically valid. It should be written in a way that any staff member would understand its meaning.

Indicators may be structure, process, or outcome in origin. The organization's ability to provide quality patient care, for example, resources, equipment, and qualification of professionals, is expressed as a structure indicator. Process indicators evaluate the way in which care is delivered, for example, assessment and patient teaching. Results of care, for example, complications, adverse reactions, and customer satisfaction are known as outcome indicators.

In keeping with the concept of continuous improvement and focusing on the process of care, indicators are developed by a representative of the staff who is involved with the activity or function. The team may involve those members within the nursing arena or members from several departments. With this approach the indicators will be defined by the "experts" or those most knowledgeable about the aspect of care. By cooperatively working together, decrease in duplication and conservation of resources are accomplished.

Sentinel and rate-based events are two types of indicators.[3] A serious, undesirable process or outcome of care, for example, death of a normal newborn, is referred to as a sentinel event. This type of indicator normally does not occur frequently but requires investigation each time it occurs because of its impact on the patient, family, or the organization. Rate-based indicators measure care during a period of time, that is, normal appendix rate. Individual review is required if the rate exceeds a predetermined rate (threshold) or a significant trend. In establishing rate indicators, great importance must be placed on identifying the appropriate numerator and denominator. Otherwise, the data would not be valid. The numerator is the number of patients to whom the event occurred, whereas the denominator is the number of patients who have the condition or procedure the indicator is assessing, for example, normal appendix divided by all appendectomies minus incidental appendectomies.

Step 5: Establish Threshold for Evaluation

There are two fundamental approaches to evaluating quality. The first is the establishment of a threshold for evaluation or an acceptability level. Threshold for evaluation is a predetermined level or point in the cumulative data analysis that triggers the need for further evaluation. For sentinel events the threshold is 0% or 100%, for example, 0% for maternal death, whereas a rate-based threshold could be 95%, for example, initial RN assessments within 4 hours of admission.

The assignment of the actual threshold depends on the seriousness of the event, its application to quality patient care, and management's willingness to live with the consequences. As in indicator development, the team should establish the threshold based on literature, experience, past performance, or customer expectation. Threshold for evaluation should not be confused with compliance to a standard of care. Thresholds are utilized because of limited resources. For example, the standard of care for the initial assessment by a registered nurse within 4 hours of admission is 100%, whereas the threshold may be set at 95%. Management may not want to invest a large amount of time and energy to change the practice if at least 95% of the patients are assessed within the appropriate time frame.

The alternate approach to evaluating care is that quality improvement is like a spiral staircase without an end. Therefore there is no room for acceptable errors in the delivery of care, but a commitment and involvement by every staff member at every level will improve the quality of care. With this in mind, the threshold need not remain constant but should be ever-changing to strive for continual improvement.

Step 6: Collect and Organize Data

This step is by far the most time consuming for the nurse. For each identified indicator, data sources, data collection methods, sampling techniques, frequency of collection, and responsibility for collection and organization of data are identified. To prevent duplication and conserve time and energy of the data collector(s), make use of existing data sources whenever possible, for example, medical records, incident and infection reports, and departmental logs. To allow for identification of patterns, trends, problems, or opportunities for improvement across departmental lines, data collection should be comprehensive, coordinated, systematic, and integrated.

Collection of data may be performed by concurrent, retrospective, interviews, observation, or any combination of the aforementioned. Many professionals believe that retrospective reviews are easiest. Although they require more resources, they are the least effective in changing practice since the patient has been discharged from the facility. Interviews and observations are the most time consuming and expensive to the facility.

During the years, there has been much discussion relative to sampling techniques and adequate size of the sample. Probability and nonprobability are two methods worth exploring. With probability each case has an equal chance of selection for the review process. This method includes using numbers tables—stratified or systematic. Although this frightens the person unfamiliar with the terminology, it is the most scientific. Convenience, purposive, or quota sampling, which are nonprobability methods, reflect qualitative judgment. This approach does not produce a statistically valid scientific study but an adequate sample that reflects current practice based on the indicator. The latter is used in most quality assessment activities.

Step 7: Evaluate Care

Interpretation of the data is key to developing an effective action plan. According to Kerlinger, "to interpret is to explain, to find meaning."[7] The data is evaluated for patterns or trends as it is related to problems or opportunities to improve care. At this point, professional practice is compared with preestablished indicators and thresholds. In addition to examining the data for trends, the nurse should describe the findings and draw conclusions. Attention should be given to the link between process and outcome of care. One must understand the clinical decision-making process and all surrounding factors to understand how practice can be changed. The evaluation can be performed by an individual in a peer review setting or by a team. In other words, focus on the causative factors and not just on individual performance. Common causes of problems deal with system deficiencies, knowledge, behavior, and performance. The key is to determine in an objective manner the area of care needing improvement.

The difficulty arises when determining exactly how care or service can be improved. Reverting to the industrial model, many tools can be used to help teams understand the underlying causes of indicator results. The following is a brief explanation of the most common tools:

Flow charts	A flow chart graphically represents the sequence of events or steps that are required in a particular process or to produce a specific output.
Cause-and-effect diagram	The cause-and-effect diagram looks like a fishbone with the effect being the desired outcome and the causes represented by the "spines." The causes are usually divided into four categories: materials, methods, manpower, and machines. This tool is referred to as a fishbone diagram or Ishikawa, named after a leading QI authority in Japan.
Run chart	The run chart displays events or observations over time.
Pareto chart	The pareto chart displays data in a ranking order comparing factors used to determine priorities, a way to sort out the "vital few" from the "trivial many."
Histogram	The histogram displays a graphic summary of how frequently something occurs.
Control chart	The control chart distinguishes common cause and special cause variation. It appears as a run chart with statistically determined upper and lower limits above and below the average.
Scatter diagram	The scatter diagram demonstrates the relationship between two variables.

Step 8: Take Action to Improve Care

An action plan is initiated if a problem or opportunity to improve care was identified during the evaluation process. An underlying philosophy to effect change is to approach the area of concern in a positive, not punitive, way. The action must be appropriate for the problem or opportunity relative to cause, severity, and scope. The written plan must identify who or what is expected to change, who is responsible for implementing the action plan, and when the change is expected to occur. If the concern in question cannot be solved interdepartmentally or intradepartmentally, recommendations are referred to the body that has authority to act. Most often a multidisciplinary approach is indicated because nursing care interfaces with the majority of the caregivers in the organization.

Step 9: Assess Actions and Document Improvement

The only way to assess the effectiveness of an action plan is to continue to monitor and evaluate the results by using the original indicators and data collection tools. Changing the tools in midstream may skew the results. Step nine addresses the question, "did we make a difference in patient care?" If improvement is identified through follow-up, the monitoring and evaluation process is continued to document continued improvement in care. If change does not occur, reassess the problem, data, causes, and the action plan before collecting additional data. Reassessment always follows a change in the action plan.

Ongoing monitoring should continue until improvement has been maintained for a substantial time. After this period, monitoring may be planned but sporadically to check sustained improvement. The leaders may determine that other indicators such as customer satisfaction surveys may show evidence of continued improvement. In this case, previous indicators would not be used.

Step 10: Communicate Information

The monitoring and evaluation activities must be communicated to all those affected by the results. In addition, the QI activities must be reported to the facility QI program as described in the organizational plan. Documenting and communicating the findings, conclusions, recommendations, actions, and results of action by the nursing staff and other team members encourage integration of information within the structure of the overall organizational plan.

❖ WHAT IF "ALL IS WELL"?

At times the quality improvement activities may prove to be unproductive. In this case one should assess each step within the QI process. If time and thought have gone into the development phase, the scope and important aspects of care will not change from year to year unless a service has been added or deleted. If problems or opportunities are not identified, evaluate the way in which the indicators are written. They may be too broad or may not measure the important aspect of care appropriately. If this is the case, redefine the indicator. The next step is to analyze the data collection techniques as outlined under step six and make adjustments, if indicated. The key is to make it work for you by making it meaningful to you and your patients.

❖ CONFIDENTIALITY OF QUALITY ASSESSMENT ACTIVITIES

In most states quality assessment/improvement activities are protected and considered confidential. The nurse administrator and QI coordinator should explore individual state requirements because not all are the same. Some common sense approaches regarding protection of data are to maintain all QA/QI activities in a locked file, to control distribution of information, to present findings on overhead rather than in handouts, to avoid mailing QA/QI reports, to number handouts and collect them at the end of the meeting, and to document summary information in minutes with a full report retained in the QA/QI file.

❖ IMPLICATIONS FOR PRACTICE

Implications for nursing practice are many if the nurse chooses to take advantage of participating in quality improvement. First, the nurse must recognize quality as a valuable element of nursing practice. In today's health care arena the nurse is requested to do more with less. If this is true, how can change be effected with limited resources? The nurse can begin by seeking meaning in what and how things are done. Quality improvement processes allow for creativity in accomplishing goals.

The nurse must enter into a collaborative practice with other health care professionals to initiate changes in patient care. Self-satisfaction comes from knowing that the nurse has had a part in affecting the quality of care. As practiced today, quality improvement offers the nurse a challenge to learn new methodologies. QA/QI activities begin to link nursing with research in documenting those things that are important to nursing practice. Quality assessment/improvement activities can empower nurses to effect change in practice patterns. As a result of working together to improve patient care, the quality improvement process will prove to be successful and beneficial to patients.

❖ DEFINING SCOPE OF PRACTICE IN EACH NURSING AREA

An example of the overall scope of care for a department of nursing is given in Appendix 5-1. To address the scope of practice in each area of nursing, examples of aspects of care, indicators, and thresholds also are given in Appendix 5-1. The important aspect of care is identified by high risk (HR), high volume (HV), or problem-prone (PP). At the end of each indicator, the type of indicator is specified as structure, process, or outcome and the type of event is designated as sentinel or rate-based.

❖ SUMMARY

Implementation of the continuous quality improvement process is vital to the future of health care delivery. The success of QI depends on the commitment of the leaders, as well as each person providing care or services. To accomplish improvement, an integrated, team approach must be initiated. The executive must set the example by removing barriers and establishing a working relationship with all those involved in patient care.

Many positive things can result from a continuous improvement atmosphere. Nurses can be challenged to increase their knowledge to define new and different approaches to address new and old problems. Motivation and commitment to the process can lead to increased retention and the ability to attract new nursing staff. The most important of all outcomes of the QI process is an improvement in the quality of patient care.

REFERENCES

1. *Accreditation manual for hospitals, 1991*, JCAHO, Chicago, 1990.
2. Berwick D: *Curing health care: new strategies for quality improvement*, San Francisco, 1990, Jossey-Bass.
3. Characteristics of Clinical Indicators, *Qual Rev Bull* 15(11):333, JCAHO, Chicago, 1989.
4. Donabedian A: *Exploration in quality assessment and monitoring: the definition of quality and approaches to its assessment. I.* Ann Arbor, Mich, 1980, Health Administration Press.
5. *Historical summary of the Joint Commission*, JCAHO, Chicago.
6. James B: Report to the AHA, *Quality management for health care delivery*, August 1989.
7. Kerlinger RN,: Principles of analysis and interpretation, In *Foundations of behavioral research*, ed 2, New York, 1973, Holt, Rinehart & Winston.
8. *Primer on clinical indicator development and application*, JCAHO, Chicago, 1990.
9. Roberts JS, Coale JG, Redman RR: A history of the joint commission on accreditation of hospitals, *JAMA* 258(7): 939–940.
10. *Transitions: From QA to CQI*, JCAHO, Chicago, 1991.

APPENDIX 5-1

TYPES OF INDICATORS

Structure Measures the organization's ability to deliver quality patient care
Process Evaluates the way in which care is delivered
Outcome Results of care

TYPES OF EVENTS

Sentinel Serious, undesirable outcome of care requiring investigation of each event
Rate-Based Measures care over time (trend)

SCOPE OF CARE - NURSING
Activities Method

Type of Patients Served:
Type of Conditions, Diagnosis, Treatments:
Type of Services Provided:
Type and Number of Staff:
Sites of Care/Service Delivery:
Times When Care/Services Are Delivered:

SCOPE OF CARE - NURSING
Key Functions Method

Staff Availability
Medication Usage
Assessment
Planning
Teaching
Documentation
Customer Satisfaction
Infection Control
Risk Control

EXAMPLE: SCOPE OF CARE - NURSING SERVICES
Activities Method

The department of nursing services provides medical, surgical, emergency, obstetric, and newborn care to all age-groups. The major diagnoses/conditions are chest pain, acute myocardial infarction, COPD, pneumonia, normal delivery, and trauma. The major surgical/invasive procedures are cholecystectomy, open and closed reduction of fractures, hysterectomy, abdominal exploration, appendectomy, cystoscopy, colonoscopy, c-section, and tonsillectomy. Nursing care is provided by registered nurses, licensed practical nurses, certified nursing assistants, and unit secretaries on a 24-hour basis within the hospital proper.

EXAMPLE - IMPORTANT ASPECTS OF CARE
Nursing Services

1. Appropriate Levels of Professional Staff
2. Nursing Process - Assessing, Planning, Implementation, Education
3. Discharge Planning
4. Management of the Obstetric Patient
5. Management of the Critically Ill Patient
6. Management of the Surgical Patient
7. Management of the Geriatric Patient
8. Management of the Medical Patient
9. Safety
10. Infection Control

MEDICAL NURSING

Aspect of Care: Patient Safety (HR) (PP)
Indicator/Threshold: All four side rails will be maintained in the up position on patients receiving medication for pain or sleep as evidenced by documentation in the nurses' notes at least every shift. (95%) (PROCESS) (RATE-BASED)

SURGICAL NURSING

Aspect of Care: Management of the Postoperative Patient (HV)
Indicator/Threshold: Mortality related to postoperative nosocomial pneumonia. (0%) (OUTCOME) (SENTINEL)

OBSTETRIC NURSING

Aspect of Care: Management of the Patient Receiving Pitocin (HR) (PP)
Indicator/Threshold: Pitocin shall be administered by the approved protocol. (100%) (PROCESS) (SENTINEL)
Aspect of Care: Management of the Newborn with Hyperbilirubinemia (HR) (PP)
Indicator/Threshold: Protective pads will be maintained on all newborns placed under the bili-light. (100%) (PROCESS)

OPERATING ROOM

Aspect of Care: Management of the Patient in Postoperative Holding (HR) (HV)
Indicator/Threshold: Patients remaining in postoperative holding for more than 1 ½ hours because of complications, for example, difficulty breathing, difficulty in recovering from anesthesia, effects of pain medication. (0%) (OUTCOME) (SENTINEL)

AMBULATORY CARE

Aspect of Care: (AMBULATORY SURGERY) Patient Education (HV) (PP)
Indicator/Threshold: Patient shall verbalize understanding of education relative to his or her procedure as evidenced by documentation and signature of the patient/significant other. (95%) (PROCESS) (RATE-BASED)
Aspect of Care: (AMBULATORY DAY CLINIC) Management of the Diabetic Patient (HV) (PP)
Indicator/Threshold: 1. The nurse shall teach the patient to prepare insulin for administration on the first visit. (98%) (PROCESS) (RATE-BASED)
2. The patient shall demonstrate understanding by a return demonstration of insulin administration on the second visit. (98%) (PROCESS) (RATE-BASED)
3. Unplanned admissions to the hospital because of complications of insulin administration. (0%) (OUTCOME) (SENTINEL)

EMERGENCY SERVICES

Aspect of Care: Assessment—Triage (HV) (HR)
Indicator/Threshold: All patients will be assessed by a triage registered

nurse within 5 minutes of arrival. (99%) (PROCESS) (RATE-BASED)

SPECIAL CARE UNIT

Aspect of Care: Management of Patient with Chest Tubes (HR)
Indicator/Threshold: 1. Physical assessment of chest and chest tube drainage every 2 hours. (98%) (PROCESS) (RATE-BASED)
2. Intake and output assessed every 8 hours. (98%) (PROCESS) (RATE-BASED)
3. Reoccurring atelectasis (0%) (OUTCOME) (SENTINEL)

LONG-TERM CARE SERVICES

Aspect of Care: Management of Nutritional Status (HV) (PP)
Indicator/Threshold: The patient's weight shall not vary more than 5 pounds each month. (0%) (OUTCOME) (SENTINEL)

HOME HEALTH SERVICES

Aspect of Care: Appropriate staff levels (HV) (HR) (PP)
Indicator/Threshold: All professional staff members shall have a current, valid license to practice within their area of expertise. (100%) (STRUCTURE) (SENTINEL)

PSYCHIATRIC SERVICES

Aspect of Care: Management of the Suicidal Patient (HR) (PP)
Indicator/Threshold: All patients shall be assessed for suicidal tendencies within 1 hour of admission and every 8 hours as long as the patient exhibits suicidal tendencies. (100%) (PROCESS) (RATE-BASED)

SUBSTANCE ABUSE SERVICES

Aspect of Care: Management during the Detoxification Period (HR) (HV)
Indicator/Threshold: Blood pressure, pulse, and respirations will be assessed every 15 minutes during the first 8 hours of admission. (95%) (PROCESS) (RATE-BASED)

CHAPTER 6

Utilization Management

❖ INTRODUCTION

Utilization management in health care can be defined as a series of actions to produce a quality health care product in a cost-effective manner while contributing to the overall goals of an institution. Utilization management seeks to identify and resolve problems that can result in excessive resource utilization and inefficient care delivery. Utilization management is a critical component of an integrated quality management process and the key to a successful quality assessment process.

Utilization review includes assessment, the process whereby the reviewer assesses the use of professional care, services, and procedures, and evaluation of the need and appropriateness of care. Utilization review intervenes and proposes solutions for situations in which cost and quality are jeopardized and screens patients for discharge needs and follow-up care.

Historically factors that contribute to utilization problems are lack of incentives for controlling costs, lack of actual cost awareness by medical and professional staff, non-individualized care such as ordering diagnostic tests out of habit, lack of community resources, and ineffective scheduling of tests or services.

❖ THE HISTORICAL BASIS OF UTILIZATION MANAGEMENT

The discovery of antibiotics, increased access to care, and government support of health care research created a highly technical and sophisticated system of health care in the United States. As the system evolved, the health of the overall population improved and the cost steadily increased. Fees for

> **TEFRA 1982**
>
> - Set pay incentives for costs below a targeted level
> - Replaced PSRO with PRO
> - Required hospitals to release information to the PRO
> - Required hospitals to implement quality assurance and utilization review programs

services were established by individual providers of care and institutions. Once services were rendered, claims were filed and payments made. There were no restrictions on what services were rendered or what charges were billed.

In 1965 Congress passed legislation creating Medicare and Medicaid that guaranteed health care to the elderly, indigent, and permanently disabled. This was the first government-funded health care package and created a larger market for health care services. Further expansion of the health care market was seen as organ transplantation became more common and surgical techniques were refined. Longevity increased for those once believed incurable or terminal. For-profit health care flourished, and government funds were allocated to build hospitals.

By 1970 the federal government was paying approximately 40% of all hospital expenditures. The increasing cost of care and increasing numbers of persons covered by Medicare and Medicaid led the government to devise mechanisms to control cost. In response, legislation was passed in 1972 that created the Professional Standards Review Organization (PSRO). The PSRO employed physician reviewers whose role was to review medical records of Medicare patients for quality, medical need, and appropriateness of the setting. In 1974 the Department of Health, Education, and Welfare (HEW) released a utilization review standard to further define resource utilization.

The Tax Equity and Fiscal Responsibility Act (TEFRA) was passed by Congress in 1982. It provided pay incentives to hospitals for holding costs below a target level and repealed the PSRO, replacing it with the Peer Review Organization (PRO). TEFRA required hospitals to release information to the PRO regarding hospital stays and to establish quality and utilization review programs (see Box above).

The PRO had responsibilities to the Health Care Financing Administra-

> **PRO Responsibilities to HCFA**
>
> Assure that:
> - hospital services were reasonable and necessary
> - care met professionally recognized standards of care
> - services were provided in most economical setting
> - patients received accurate bills for diagnosis and procedures
>
> Recommend sanctions

tion to determine that Medicare patients received hospital services that were reasonable and necessary and that care met professionally recognized standards of care. The PRO was responsible to see that services were provided in the most economically appropriate setting and that patients received accurate bills for diagnoses and procedures (see Box above).

As part of the contractual arrangement with the PRO, hospitals were required to inform Medicare patients in writing that their hospital admission and care might be reviewed by the PRO and request prior PRO approval for readmissions. Hospitals were required to advise the PRO when notice was given to a patient whose admission to or continued stay was determined medically unnecessary for an inpatient setting. Finally, hospitals were required to accept financial responsibility for all care that was determined medically unnecessary.

In 1983 amendments to the Social Security Act, Title VI, added rules for the implementation of PROs. In 1974 the government accepted bids from review organizations that wanted to become peer review organizations. Many that applied were old PSROs. Geographic boundaries were set to coincide with state or regional boundaries. PRO performance would be monitored, and they would not be allowed to delegate review to other organizations. Confidentiality had to be maintained, and information shared had to be used only to carry out official functions. Hospitals were required to contract with a PRO, and sanctions could be recommended by the PRO, including withholding payment.

Title VI of the Social Security amendment created the prospective pricing system (PPS). Under PPS, payment for care was based on a predetermined price. Limits for determining cost were based on calculations of routine nursing costs for each diagnosis.

> ### Title VI Social Security Amendment Expansion PRO Review
>
> - Admission and preadmission review
> - Outlier review
> - Invasive procedure review
> - DRG validation

> ### Title VI Social Security Amendment
>
> - Created prospective pricing system
> - Based reimbursement for care on predetermined fixed price based on nursing costs
> - Established deadlines for implementing the prospective pricing system
> - Expanded PRO review and clarified functions

Title VI expanded PRO review and clarified PRO functions. Functions included admission and preadmission review, which determined need for admission before or on admission. Outlier review involved the review of cases in which cost for inpatient stay was greater than the predetermined amount when inpatient days exceeded the expected number. PROs were required to review patients who had undergone an invasive procedure and to validate diagnoses submitted for pay (see Box above). Before Title VI, hospitals were responsible for quality review. PRO was now given that responsibility. From the inception of the PRO in 1982 until the present, the government has continually refined the PRO functions. The First Scope of Work for the PRO was from 1985-1986 and the Second Scope of Work covered 1987-88. The Third Scope of Work is based on extensive analyses of the Second Scope of Work and incorporated provisions of COBRA law of 1985 and OBRA of 1986 and 1987. Review procedures for the PRO program have become more standardized with the 1989-1992 Third Scope of Work.

The Home Care Quality Improvement (HCQI) Act was passed in 1986. This act provided immunity from monetary damages for persons providing peer review activities, that is, the PRO, on other practitioners. This immunity was granted provided the peer review action was performed to further high-quality care, taking into consideration all information available.

> ### PRO Enforcement Mechanisms
>
> - Impose education on hospital staff
> - Can change DRG assignment if disagreement with facility
> - Can report problems to HCFA or the Office of Inspector General (OIG)
> - Deny payment entire hospital stay
> - Fine the institution
> - Exclude institutions from providing care to Medicare institutions
> - Publish facility in local paper listing violation and sanction imposed or effective date and duration of the exclusion from Medicare program

This law gave hospitals and physicians the opportunity for full consideration before the PRO sent a letter to the patient, stating that the hospitals stay would not be covered. HCQI established a new federal agency to research the effectiveness and appropriateness of various PRO procedures and to provide guidelines to providers. HCQI guaranteed a safeguard for PROs in the performance of what government was mandating a PRO to do in records review and protected them against repercussions for following enforcement mechanisms.

Diagnostic related groups (DRGs) were originally developed in the 1960s as a patient classification system. Yale University researchers John Thompson and Robert Fletcher refined the system in 1975 by using statistical techniques to determine patients who were likely to become inpatients with similar number of inpatient days and services. The groupings of days or length of stay norms were based on 23 major diagnostic categories (MDCs) based on major organ systems.

PPS was based on a DRG system. Payment under PPS was predetermined or capitated. Some allowance was made for complications, but payment was basically fixed. When PPS was introduced, 50% of all hospital inpatients had Medicare coverage. Therefore one half of hospital revenue was based on DRGs and PPS and on a capitated payment. Hospitals began to experience more difficulty in producing revenue and were heavily scrutinized by the PRO. The PRO was empowered to impose punishments and could deny payment for overutilization of medical care and for practices deemed by the PRO to be of poor quality (Box above describes PRO enforcement).

> ### Utilization Management Program Components
>
> - Written plan
> - Communication mechanisms with medical and professional staff
> - Interface with PRO
> - Review activities based on physician-approved objective criteria
> - Systems development to identify problem areas
> - Mechanisms for collecting, analyzing, and reporting data
> - Knowledge of laws and reimbursement
> - Physician advisor

❖ UTILIZATION MANAGEMENT PROGRAM CREATION

The capitated payment system and increased scrutiny by the PRO with the potential for punitive consequences forced hospitals to create a means by which practices of care providers and institutions could be monitored. In response, hospitals began developing their own utilization management programs. The focus of these programs was to ensure that patients received the care needed in the most appropriate setting based on diagnosis and presenting condition. Programs were designed to evaluate professional medical care, services, and procedures against a predetermined criteria and the facility as a whole. Federal regulations dictated utilization review for Medicare patients, and UR guidelines for Medicaid recipients were provided by individual states.

Program development in hospitals included a written plan of utilization review and mechanisms to interact with medical and professional staffs on patients with UR issues. Utilization management programs typically dealt with PRO denials of payment for perceived poor quality or overuse of resources and performed review activities much like the PRO, based on objective criteria approved by medical staff. Utilization management programs developed systems for identifying problem cases, practitioners, departments or services, and mechanisms for collecting, analyzing, and reporting data. Knowledge of laws and regulations and reimbursement or payor practices provided a basis for overall UR activities. Physical-related issues concerning quality utilization or liability are referred to the physician advisor for review. (see Box above for components of a utilization management program).

> ### Utilization Management Activities Acute Care
>
> Assessment
>   Admissions
>   Level of care
>   Resource use
>   Need for continued stay
>   Discharge
> Evaluation
>   Overutilization
>   Underutilization
>   Inefficiencies
>   Lack of cost restraint
> Intervention
>   Problems adversely affecting cost and quality
> Discharge planning
>   Identifying needs after patient leaves hospital

> ### Utilization Management Activities Outpatient Setting
>
> Assess
>   Continuity of care per illness
>   Patient/family ability to follow plan
>   Postdischarge needs

❖ UTILIZATION MANAGEMENT ACTIVITIES

Basic utilization management activities in acute care include review and assessment of the use of professional care, services, and procedures for need and appropriateness. In evaluation of need and appropriateness, staff members look for patterns of overutilization and underutilization of services, as well as inefficiencies in scheduling and lack of cost containment. UR intervenes in areas in which problems are identified that adversely affect the balance between cost effectiveness and quality and also works with discharge planning to identify a patient's needs after leaving the hospital (see Box above).

In the outpatient setting, utilization management seeks to assess the patient's continuity of care needs through a period of illness and patient and family ability and willingness to follow their treatment plan. Utilization management also provides input on referrals and access to available community resources (see Box on p. 79).

❖ VARIOUS APPROACHES TO REVIEW

Utilization management programs utilize a variety of techniques and approaches to monitor care. Prospective review involves review of proposed care related to level of care and setting. Financial assessment is made to determine the patient's ability to pay for the treatment proposed.

Concurrent review determines the need and appropriateness of care on admission or within 24 hours. The need for continued stay is assessed at specified intervals throughout a hospital stay by reviewing use of ancillary services such as laboratory, x-ray, and level of care. Criteria used in concurrent and continued stay are normative or empirical. Normative are based on the opinion of professionals; empirical are based on actual practice of professionals.

Retrospective review is done after a patient is discharged from the hospital. In retrospective review the reviewer gets an overall picture of the hospital stay, and patient outcomes and cost can be compared. Funds and practice patterns are more easily identified in retrospective review.

Focused review focuses on singular issues and is often based on what the PRO reviews. Focused review is very specific, with case selections based on internally identified problems or outside agency requests (see Box below).

Review Types

Concurrent
    Medical necessity and appropriateness in admission and continued stay
Retrospective
    Complete hospital stay reviewed after patient is discharged
Focused
    Review focuses on specific issue, often what PRO is reviewing
Prospective
    Review of proposed care before care delivery
    Financial assessment of proposed care

❖ UTILIZATION MANAGEMENT CRITERIA

Criteria that will be used in the review process should be developed by utilization management staff and preapproved by the medical staff to meet the needs of the institution. Use of criteria is an attempt to establish the medical need for admission as an inpatient and the appropriateness and need for specific types of care, procedures, treatments, and readiness for discharge. Using the criteria, the utilization management staff compares all documented patient signs, symptoms, complaints, previous diagnoses, test results, treatment, and other available data.

Documentation of nonspecific diagnoses, vague complaints, and systems is discussed with the attending physician, physician advisor, or both. The medical staff has an overall responsibility to act on physician-related utilization management problems. Intervention may be done with the physician advisor through a committee such as a utilization review committee or a medical executive committee. Administration is responsible for intervention when utilization problems are attributable to the hospital and the staff (see Box below).

❖ CRITERIA SYSTEMS

Diagnosis specific review criteria involve the use of the physician's history and physical and the emergency room record. There are two distinct steps required in justifying admission. Using the criteria, the reviewer verifies that a specific condition exists and validates the need for inpatient admission.

Severity of illness/intensity of service criteria make up a generic system used in many acute care facilities. Criteria are divided into major body systems and can be used on admission and throughout inpatient stay. Documentation of clinical findings is used to assign severity. Intensity of service refers to prescribed medical care that can be provided only in a hospital setting.

Criteria Systems

- Diagnosis specific review
- Severity of illness/intensity of service
- Length of stay
- Appropriateness evaluation protocol
- Normative/empirical criteria

Length of stay criteria are based on the data of patients with specific conditions and the number of days spent as an inpatient. Factors such as age, single or multiple diagnoses, or surgeries are compiled and then aggregated as numbers of inpatient days. Norms are based on data in regions. Length of normal stay should not be used as the only guideline but should be balanced against clinical criteria.

The appropriateness evaluation protocol (AEP) is a criteria system used for adult medical/surgical patients. Two appropriateness decisions based on medical records information are made. If any of the criteria is met, the admission is considered appropriate. Day appropriateness is determined when a patient meets criteria in either of three subsets: medical service, nursing/life support, or patient condition factors.

Normative or empirical criteria are used in concurrent and continued stay review. Normative criteria are based on the opinion of professionals; empirical criteria are based on the actual practice of professionals.

❖ MANAGEMENT OF UTILIZATION MANAGEMENT DATA

Utilization management programs are required to have a plan with stated program objectives and screening criteria. A program must employ efficient mechanisms for physician referral to a physician advisor or UR committees to review and advise on questionable cases. Efficient and accurate data collection is essential, as well as review of quality assessment data for trends in departments, services, or practitioners. Good intradepartmental communication is helpful in making referrals to groups such as social service, risk management, infection control, and discharge planning. Good communication is also positive when departments or services collaborate on patient care needs, issues, or concerns.

❖ PATIENT CLASSIFICATION SYSTEMS

Patient classification systems are a means by which patient conditions are classified. Classification systems are used for utilization management, quality and risk management, institutional planning and management, and reimbursement financial divisions of institutions.

A diagnostic related group (DRG) is a patient classification system selected by HCFA for the Medicare prospective pricing system. The DRG payment categorizes and pays the average cost for illnesses that have similar characteristics. The DRG system surmised that hospital cases could be

grouped into clinical classifications that had similar resource usage. DRGs did not take into account persons with advanced disease. DRG assignment for a patient is based on the following:
1. Principal diagnosis
2. Principal procedure, if any
3. Complications
4. Comorbidities
5. Age

Principal diagnosis is the condition that is largely responsible for causing the admission of the patient to the hospital. *Principal procedure* refers to the procedure performed for treatment that is most closely related to the principal diagnosis. *Provisional diagnosis* is the preliminary or admitting diagnosis, the condition before study that caused the inpatient admission. *Comorbidity* is expected in 75% of cases to increase the length of stay by at least 1 day. Of the 475 DRG numbers, only one may be assigned per hospitalization. The DRG numbers fluctuate annually.

DRG information can provide data on problems for utilization management. In the form of case mix information, data can be obtained on DRGs losing money, DRGs consuming most ancillary services such as x-ray and lab, and physician treatment patterns.

❖ CASE MIX

Case mix index is a combination of clinical and financial information. Case mix information includes types and ages of patients and types of service and disease groups. The DRG system is a type of case mix classification system. Data services for case mix systems include the patient's medical record, bill, patient acuity reports, and any available severity level indexes. Case mix is a combination of clinical and financial information but is based on charge data rather than actual cost.

Case mix is affected by demographics, services offered, hospital and physician referrals, specialty composition of medical staff, and patient distribution across diagnostic and procedural categories.

❖ REIMBURSEMENT/THIRD-PARTY PAYORS

Prospective payment is a charge-based system that pays hospitals and providers a fixed set of payment rates for each type of patient. The payment rate remains the same regardless of actual cost. The objective of this payment system is to reduce cost and improve the operating efficiency of the institution and care provider. Physicians are expected to administer the most efficient plan of treatment while maintaining quality. The DRG system is used by Medicare and some Blue Cross plans. Other federal reimbursement systems include CHAMPUS, which is a health care insurance program for civilians in government service, Veterans Administration, and Medicaid for indigent, elderly, and disabled in which payment limits are determined by the state. Private insurance companies have joined the federal government in cost-containment efforts. Many employ techniques similar to those used by the government, such as precertifying, performing their own utilization review, and capitating payments.

❖ CASE MANAGEMENT

Case management is a means of coordinating and integrating all phases of patient care/determining available resources. Case managers generally are nurses or social workers working within the treating facility or for an employee or case management company. Case managers are concerned with the characteristics of the illness or injury, psychosocial factors such as support systems and family members, financial issues, access to available community resources, and short- and long-term goals.

Case Management Concerns

- Complexity of illness or injury
- Diagnostic and therapeutic needs
- Psychosocial factors
- Medication and equipment needs
- Support systems
- Economic issues
- Accessibility to community resources
- Motivation to get well
- Degree of incapacitation after an acute illness
- Long-term and short-term goals

❖ DISCHARGE PLANNING

Discharge planning is a multidisciplinary approach to prepare the patient for movement to another level of care or for home. Discharge planning centers on patient needs, as well as family support. The discharge plan may be to move the patient to self-care, care of family or significant other, or by an organized provider of care such as long-term care, rehabilitation units, or home health care. Discharge planning is critical to utilization management. The Joint Commission has approved standards requiring hospitalwide policies and procedures for discharge planning, and discharge planning is a required component of the utilization management plan. The Joint Commission standard for discharge planning delineates the role of the physician or licensed practitioner responsible for the patient, the nursing, social service, and other support staff, and the patient, the patient's family, or guardian.

The Omnibus Budget Reconciliation Act (OBRA), which was passed in 1986, dictated that patients be identified at the beginning of hospitalization for those likely to have adverse health on discharge, if there was no discharge plan. OBRA legislated timely intervention to establish a plan and required documentation of posthospital needs.

❖ JOINT COMMISSION AND UTILIZATION AND DISCHARGE PLANNING

The Joint Commission requires that hospitals provide for the utilization management program. The first Joint Commission standard was introduced in 1980. The standards require hospitals to provide for and demonstrate use of resources through a utilization management program. Utilization programs are expected to aid hospitals in providing high cost quality care by addressing overutilization, underutilization, and inefficient use of resources. More specifically, JCAHO requires an organization to examine the findings of quality assessment activities and results of patient care studies and review surgical cases, drug usage, and blood utilization.

❖ UTILIZATION AND QUALITY ASSESSMENT

Utilization management is integral to and greatly dependent on an effective quality assessment program. Utilization management attempts to determine at what point quality might be compromised as hospitals look to contain costs. Quality assessment data is often used to review ancillary services and practitioners.

❖ UNDER/OVERUTILIZATION

Underutilization of resources is a serious impediment of quality care. Underordering of resources such as diagnostic tests and drugs, although initially reducing cost, will likely cost the patient, facility, and care provider over time. If treatment or diagnostics are underordered, patient illnesses may lengthen, which causes increased pain and suffering, as well as residual damage. That decreases patient productivity, which could result in institutionalization or even death. Quality is also compromised when underutilization results in prolonged physician care or need for rehabilitation. Prolonged illnesses because of underutilization will create financial concerns for the patient and family. Underutilization can affect the speed with which health problems are detected and treatment initiated.

Overutilization can be equally as detrimental. Any test or procedure creates a potential for an adverse occurrence or a bad outcome. Therefore overordering of tests, medications, and treatments can create a potentially harmful environment. Overutilization may create financial burdens. Overutilization of resources can decrease the viability of the institution under capitated payment systems.

❖ EXAMPLES OF UTILIZATION MANAGEMENT IN DIFFERENT SETTINGS

Regardless of setting, utilization management serves to ensure quality, cost-contained health care. Although the basic objective remains the same, the issues at different levels of care vary. In the acute care setting, utilization management reviews the need for admission, continued stay, reasonableness of care, and appropriateness for discharge to home or other care. Utilization management in long-term care also addresses admission need but looks to see if long-range goals are evident as a preparation for outcomes such as future discharge. Resource utilization such as the use of laboratory or x-ray diagnostics would be reviewed as in acute care. In an outpatient diagnostic center, utilization management could review appropriateness of setting and timeliness and scheduling of services. Inefficient scheduling could increase cost and delay needed diagnostics or care.

The collaboration of nursing and utilization management enhances the quality of patient care. When working together, staff members can address issues concurrently to ensure that patients receive timely, appropriate care. Discharge planning is enhanced through a team approach. Through the use of nursing process and constant contact with patients, nurses have a unique position to be a superb data source for patient information, departments, services, physicians, and family members. Nursing documentation and care planning are also great data sources. Nurses can serve as liaisons to the multidisciplinary team and can aid utilization management in networking with medical and professional staff. Utilization management can teach professional and medical staff as reimbursement changes and give updates on PRO review criteria and insurance requirements. Working as a team promotes efficiency and quality and decreases cost thereby decreasing PRO intervention and potential lost revenue.

From a nursing perspective, working with utilization management can enhance nursing practice related to quality of patient care. Nursing serves as a hub from which care is planned and provided. Improved quality and appropriateness of care influence patient outcomes in a positive way. Collaboration with positive outcomes serves to enhance overall nursing satisfaction and is a catalyst in continued collaboration and team effort that nurses have the ability to establish.

❖ UTILIZATION MANAGEMENT AND CONTINUOUS QUALITY IMPROVEMENT (CQI)

The nurse/patient relationship can be a driving force in patient recovery. A positive rapport built on trust and a nurse's ability to educate and motivate can speed the recovery process. Consequently, resource utilization and cost will decrease. Additional effects may be a shorter length of stay and reduced readmissions, which are components of utilization management.

Utilization management is one component of an integrated quality management program and is a part of the quality assessment process. Continuous quality improvement seeks to meet customer needs, minimize dissatisfaction with services or products, avoid costly deficiencies, and optimize company performance. In continuous improvement, quality planning involves determining customer needs, developing products to meet needs, and using a team approach.

Effective utilization management employs CQI principles, determining patient care needs, improving quality, reducing cost, and optimizing overall company performance. Utilization management, like continuous quality improvement, is a continuous process beginning on or just before admission and going through discharge. Utilization management assesses postdischarge needs to link patients to available community resources. The use of a team approach interlocking all disciplines in care planning fosters the CQI concept of partnership. Education of utilization management principles to the multidisciplinary team imparts some understanding of the complexities of health care delivery, cost, quality, and appropriateness. As a result, that understanding fosters continuous improvement efforts.

❖ ADMINISTRATIVE CONCERNS AND UTILIZATION MANAGEMENT

Administrative support and allocation of resources for utilization management are unquestionable keys to success for the program. The Health Care Financing Administration will continue to refine the PRO and design care. Reimbursement for federally funded programs and private insurances will continue to decline for inpatient care. With these considerations, hospital utilization management programs will continually need support to address patient issues and educate medical and professional staff. Quality will continue to be a concern, and there will be the potential for lost revenues and decreased financial viability for institutions.

When care is linked to resource utilization, DRG data, and decreased hospital stays, a downward trend of inpatient admissions will result. Lowering censuses means a reduction in jobs and/or decreased hours. Small hospitals have the greatest risk for not surviving under these conditions. It is extremely difficult to maintain a stable professional staff when scheduling is variable based on patient census. These problems are a by-product of effective utilization and will continue to be an administrative nightmare.

Lack of physician education and hostility toward the "system" will continue to be problems as physicians are more restricted in their practice. Physicians will have to be educated and encouraged to follow established utilization guidelines. An inability to follow through will result only in quality problems, PRO and private insurance intervention by payment denial, and other punitive mechanisms. The final results will be decreased or questionable institutional viability. Physicians must have administrative support and must be encouraged to comply with the program.

Health care entities will be forced by financial implications of care to look for alternative care scenarios. Acute care is shrinking, and other means must be developed to generate revenue.

Public perception of cost and quality will also be an administrative concern. The perceptions will influence patients in their choice of where their care will be provided. Administration will want to support utilization efforts to help promote a positive image of cost and quality.

❖ SUMMARY

Utilization management is a critical component of quality management. Federal funding of Medicare and Medicaid under a cost-based health care delivery system leads to tremendous financial outlay by the federal government. An attempt to control increasing costs created the PSRO, then the PRO, to monitor cost and quality, and established PPS based on DRGs. The Joint Commission later required utilization management programs in hospitals.

Effective utilization management programs use a multidisciplinary approach enlisting the medical and professional staffs in an effort to provide care that is cost effective and appropriate for the patient. Administrative support for utilization management programs is critical to acceptance by the medical staff, which realizes that this is essential to continued viability. Improved utilization of resources will mean decreased inpatient admissions. Small institutions will have the most to lose because stable staffing will be a problem.

Finally, health care entities will need to continually look for other types of health care scenarios to provide patient care and generate income as inpatient acute care days decrease.

REFERENCES

1. Barrocas, A, Barrocas, N: Healthcare in the nineties: Old wine in new bottles, South Med J 81(2):26, 1988.
2. Brown, JA: The 1990 quality assurance professionals study guide, *Managed Care Consultant*, 1990.
3. Crocker, L, Charney, C, Chew, J S: *Quality circles a guide to participation and productivity*, New York, 1984, Hudson Books.
4. Juran JM: *Juran on leadership and quality, an executive handbook*, New York, 1989, Macmillan.
5. Kilber, P: *The national association of quality assurance professionals, quality assurance and risk management, a study guide and primer*, 1989, National Association for Health Care Quality.
6. Mid South Foundation for Medical Care, *Tennessee Peer Review Organization Provider Manual*, April 1, 1989.
7. Walton M: *The Deming management model*, New York, 1986, The Putnam Publishing Group.

CHAPTER

7

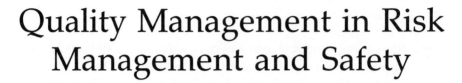

Quality Management in Risk Management and Safety

Terrye Maclin Fairly
Deborah G. Nance

❖ INTRODUCTION TO RISK MANAGEMENT/SAFETY

Risk management programs are relatively new to the health care setting. These programs have been in place in the blue collar industry since early in the nineteenth century. In the mid-1960s the concept of risk management did not exist in health care institutions. Most facilities had a safety officer, but the concentration of these efforts focused on accident prevention for employees and, to a much lesser extent, for patients and visitors. For health services that common thread is called risk management. As the law of worker's compensation and product and general liability developed and expanded, industries began to experience losses beyond the traditional casualty claims associated with weather, fire, and other events. Insurance companies expanded the scope of coverage for accidents to patients and visitors and encouraged management of the businesses to offer safety programs designed to prevent accidents. From this point risk management evolved. Incentive programs were offered by the insurance companies for organizations to have their own internal risk management programs rather than employ outside consultants.

❖ THE EMERGENCE OF HEALTH CARE RISK MANAGEMENT

During the late 1960s and early 1970s, health care began to experience a tremendous escalation in medical malpractice claims. Because of the increased frequency and severity of these claims, many insurance companies increased their premiums to astronomic amounts or stopped writing malpractice coverage all together. The response of the insurance companies was a result of their inability to predict the frequency that claims could be expected and the cost of the claim very often exceeded the premium. Studies were conducted during the early 1970s to help determine the extent of the crisis and attempt to identify some solutions. During the Nixon Administration, the Department of Health, Education, and Welfare was commissioned to conduct one of the first major studies on medical malpractice. The commission's purpose was to identify and evaluate the causes of malpractice claims, the effectiveness of professional liability insurance, the effectiveness of the legal mechanisms for compensating injured parties, and the attitude exhibited by the general public. Results of the commission revealed that malpractice claims were primarily the result of injuries or adverse consequences of medical treatment. The commission also found that not all injuries were a result of negligence or were preventable in every case. One major finding was that the severity of the injury was more likely to be the deciding factor as to whether a claim would be made against an institution. The commission also found that the most effective way to reduce the frequency and severity of injuries was to develop a medical injury prevention program in every health care setting. A study conducted in 1977 by the American Bar Association Commission on Medical Professional Liability stated that it was imperative to reduce the frequency and severity of avoidable accidents with resultant injury to patients. This study showed that in most hospitals the safety programs were aimed at improving the physical environment and were not focused on medically caused injury. This commission made the recommendation that the medical profession and health care industry work collaboratively in developing mechanisms to prevent avoidable medically related injury to patients.

The Committee on Law and Medicine of the Bar Association of the City of New York performed a study and recommended that hospitals (1) establish a medical injury prevention program, (2) focus on the investigation of causes of injuries, and (3) develop mechanisms to minimize results. Most hospitals did develop prevention programs.

❖ GOVERNMENT/INSURANCE RESPONSE TO THE MALPRACTICE CRISIS

State governments responded to the malpractice crisis by passage of legislation designed to establish limits on the amounts of awards by setting up arbitration panels. These laws proved unsuccessful because most were challenged on the grounds of unconstitutionality and thus were short lived. The insurance companies responded to the crisis by devising alternative risk financing mechanisms. These included programs such as joint underwriting. Many of these mechanisms are used today.

❖ UNDERLYING CAUSES OF INCREASED LIABILITY CLAIMS

There are a variety of reasons for the increase in health care liability claims. Increased technologic advances carry increased risk of injury, and there is an increased likelihood of errors because of the larger numbers of persons caring for patients in a facility. There is heightened awareness by the public on health care because of marketing campaigns and often a deterioration in the physician-patient relationship. Patients are often unrealistic in their expectations of their care and results of that care.

❖ THE SECOND MALPRACTICE CRISIS

The second malpractice crisis occurred in the 1980s. The overruling of many of the state laws to control malpractice claims and the influx of a great number of attorneys in the liability market caused yet another crisis. The primary effect of this crisis was a gradual increase in premiums, as well as an increase in the number and size of losses particularly in the area of obstetrics and gynecology. The insurance for this specialty remains available but is extremely costly. Thus many physicians no longer provide these services.

❖ RISK MANAGEMENT DEFINED

Risk management is one of the specialties within the general field of management. *Management* may be defined as the process of planning, organizing, leading, and controlling the resources and activities of an organization to fulfill its objectives most cost effectively.

An organization has one or more of a variety of objectives: profit, growth, public service, or the performance of a governmental function, to name a few. To achieve these objectives, an organization must first reach a more fundamental goal—survival in the face of potentially crippling accidental losses. Beyond mere survival, the top management of an organization also may wish to prevent any accidental losses from interrupting the organization's operations, which would slow its growth or reduce its profits or cash flows.

Risk management, which occupies an important place in the broad definition of management, is devoted to minimizing the adverse effects of accidental loss on the organization. Given the focus on accidental losses, *risk management,* as a managerial or administrative process, may be defined as the process of planning, organizing, leading, and controlling the activities of an organization to minimize the adverse effects of accidental losses on that organization at reasonable cost. This definition stresses the managerial aspects of risk management—what it has in common with all other forms of management in carrying out decisions with respect to potential accidental losses.

Risk management is a decision sequence for the following:
1. Identifying exposures to accidental loss that may interfere with an organization's basic objectives
2. Examining feasible alternative risk management techniques for dealing with these exposures
3. Selecting the apparently best risk management technique(s)
4. Implementing the chosen risk management technique(s)
5. Monitoring the results of the chosen technique(s) to ensure that the risk management program remains effective

These two partial definitions of risk management, one emphasizing its managerial aspects and the other emphasizing its decisional aspects, can be unified into a single definition; *risk management* is the process of making and carrying out decisions that will minimize the adverse effects of accidental losses on an organization. Making these decisions requires the five steps in the decision process. Carrying out these decisions requires the risk management professional to perform, or to guide other administrative and support staff to perform, the four functions in the management process.

The risk management process is both repetitive and self-reinforcing. It is repetitive because past choices of risk management techniques must be continually reevaluated in light of changes in an organization's activities and resulting loss exposures, changes in the relative costs of alternative risk management techniques, changes in legal requirements, and perhaps even changes in an organization's basic objectives. The risk management decision process also is self-reinforcing because its fifth step—monitoring to see if the previously selected risk management techniques have produced their expected results—will reveal the need to revise decisions when a significant change in conditions, such as in exposures, relative risk management costs, legal requirements, or an organization's objectives, causes the risk management program to fall short of its goal. This reassessment typically returns to the first step of the risk management decision process—identifying and analyzing loss exposures.

❖ IDENTIFYING AND ANALYZING LOSS EXPOSURES

The first step in risk management as a decision process is to identify and analyze loss exposures. In this context, *identifying* means to recognize the possibility of loss and to understand what accidental losses possibly could occur. *Analyze* means to estimate the likely significance of these possible losses. The significance of a loss exposure increases as the actual losses from that exposure (1) become more frequent, (2) become more severe, and/or (3) interfere more substantially with an organization's ability to achieve its objectives.

Identifying and analyzing loss exposures is the most important step in the risk management decision process because an unrecognized loss exposure cannot be intelligently managed. Once an exposure has been identified and analyzed, however, the broad outlines of how best to manage it often become immediately apparent. Like any art, exposure identification and analysis requires imagination and insight. Recognizing exposures requires the ability to visualize how particular sets of circumstances may cause both routine and extraordinary accidental losses. To assist in the identification and analysis of loss exposure, we will lay a two-part foundation: first, the four elements of any loss exposure will be identified: and, second, several widely used methods of exposure identification and analysis will be discussed.

The elements of any loss exposure are the following:
1. Value subject to loss
2. Peril causing loss
3. Financial consequences of the loss
4. Entity suffering the loss

Values subject to loss include property, net income, freedom from liability, and life and health (services) of key persons whose special talents are not easily replaced. Perils causing loss may be classified as natural (such as windstorm, earthquake, or flood), human (involving the actions of individuals in, for example, stealing property or behaving carelessly), and economic (such as unemployment or technologic change).

The financial consequences of loss exposures vary with the frequency and severity of actual losses. Less severe losses are usually more frequent than severe losses. Many possible entities such as an organization, its employees, its suppliers, or its customers may be adversely affected by a loss-causing event. In identifying and analyzing loss exposures, one must remain constantly aware of each of these four elements of a loss exposure. One must recognize that a change in any element alters the fundamental nature of the exposure and may also change the indicated choice of appropriate risk management technique(s).

As stated previously, exposure identification and analysis is at least as much an art as a science because it relies both on insight and imagination. To aid in the practice of this art, a number of basic methods have been developed to search for loss exposures. These methods are particularly valuable whenever the risk management professional must rely on others, who are perhaps less gifted in risk management insight, to assemble basic exposure information. These methods include standardized surveys/questionnaires, financial statement analyses, personal inspections, and consultations with experts within and outside the organization.

❖ NURSING AND THE RISK MANAGEMENT PROCESS

The concept of risk management has been used by the insurance industry since the 1950s. Insurance companies entered the premises of their clients to evaluate where potential risks were present and to advise on how to prevent injuries from those risks. A primary consideration was loss prevention. Although the insurance industry was primarily interested in the concept of preventing financial loss, health care providers have adapted the concept with some shift in emphasis to the prevention of death and disability to patients and employees resulting from preventable loss.

The risk management process is used basically to assess areas in which claims can be prevented. This process includes the identification, analysis, and treatment of risks. Claims that have already been brought may be handled by the risk manager. This management may occur as part of a self-insurance mechanism or may be done in conjunction with an outside insur-

ance company. Claims management is one element of risk management. The risk management role in claims management involves the following:
1. Settlement negotiations
2. Trial preparation
3. Witness interviews
4. Evidence preparation and depositions

A good risk management program has many components. Every health care employee plays a role in the risk management process. To be successful, each program must be individually molded to meet the needs of the institution. The background and experience of the risk manager help to determine the direction of the program. Nurses have assumed the risk manager's position in various types of health care facilities. The experienced nurse has much to offer in such a position because of his or her familiarity with direct patient care.

Some institutions have chosen people with an insurance background to direct risk management activities. If so, the financial aspects of risk management are usually emphasized, that is, what is insured and how to finance the risk. Engineering, safety, or administrative professionals may perform the risk management function in some facilities, but the nurse is most often the link between the administrative professionals and the assessment of clinical risks.

Let us explore the contribution and involvement of the professional nurse and the nursing service organization in the process of managing risks in the health care environment. Nursing as a profession provides the backbone of the health care system as it is known in the United States today. We find the nurse in every aspect of the provision of health care, ranging from the traditional acute setting to the nurse entrepreneur in independent practice. For this reason the nursing profession contributes substantially toward identifying and managing risks.

❖ HEALTH CARE RISKS IDENTIFIED

Risks involving the nursing profession in the health care environment involve four major directions:
1. Risks to the individual nurse professional
2. Risks to the health care employer
3. Risks to the patient, client, or visitor
4. Risks to the general public

The terms *malpractice* and *negligence* are often used interchangeably. *Neg-*

ligence is a more general term referring to a deviation from the acceptable standard of care that a reasonably prudent person would use in a particular set of circumstances. *Malpractice* is a more specific type of negligence, a deviation from a professional standard of care. Nurses, doctors, lawyers, and accountants are some types of professionals who may be liable for malpractice.

Risks to the Individual Nurse Professional

The nurse must understand the nursing role in the performance of professional duties. In the performance of professional duties a nurse is required to exercise the degree of care and skill that a reasonably prudent person with similar education, training, and experience would exercise under the same general conditions or circumstances. Standards of care and practice are established in a variety of ways:
1. State Nurse Practice Act
2. JCAHO
3. Internal policy and procedure
4. Community practice
5. Nationally recognized professional organizations
6. Nursing research

Rule of personal liability: The law does not permit a wrongdoer to avoid legal liability for his or her own wrongdoing even though someone else may be sued and held legally liable for the wrongful conduct in question under another rule or law. The implication for the nurse is that even though the employer may be legally liable for the action of the employees, the employee may also be held personally liable.

Examples of Ways Nurses May Prevent Violations of Practice Standards

1. Familiarize yourself with those standards and laws that govern the practice of nursing in your locality.
2. Know the policies of your facility and your scope of practice as outlined in your job description.
3. Take responsibility for the education and skills required to perform your particular responsibilities, including new or unfamiliar procedures.

4. Do not attempt to interpret unclear orders.

To summarize the nurse's responsibility in the risk management process:
1. The nurse has the legal responsibility to discharge his or her duty according to the recognized standard of care.
2. Each individual nurse is a risk manager. The nurse has the responsibility to identify and report unusual occurrences and potential risks to the proper authority.

As the nurse recognizes his or her role in the risk management process, individual liability and responsibility become clear. As the nurse protects himself or herself from liability by practicing within the standard of care, he or she does what benefits himself or herself and the profession. Those actions/decisions automatically benefit the patient and produce positive patient care, thereby benefitting the employer. Risks are automatically reduced through the professional conduct of the nurse.

Risks to the Health Care Employer

As in other industries, the health care employer is responsible for the safety of its employees and for others who frequent its premises. The health care industry is liable for items such as safety, environment, worker's compensation and unemployment, and product liability. In addition, it must protect itself from malpractice issues. Nursing service organizations and individual nurses assume a crucial role in assisting the employer in the reduction of liability.

As we have discussed, the individual nurse performs his or her duty to the patients in accordance with the acceptable standards governing the practice of nursing. This is the first and foremost way the individual can contribute to the well-being of the employer. The second way is by participating in the risk identification system, usually associated with incident reporting.

Incident reporting should be designed as a nonpunitive mechanism to report incidents that did or could have caused harm to patients, visitors, or employees. The reporting mechanism may also be used as a mechanism to identify potentially harmful situations to correct the danger before harm is done. The focus of the risk management department is to identify potential risks or opportunities to improve care and work toward improvement of care. In the event that an incident caused injury or harm, prompt notification of the risk management department allows for intervention or investigation that minimizes damages. Whether the facility promotes the risk identification and reporting process heavily or not, it is the responsibility of the individual nursing professional to use the proper reporting format to honestly report occurrences or potential risks. This may be another area in which individual accountability must take precedence over pressure from others.

The nursing department, as an organization, maintains responsibility for participating in the risk management process. As an organized department, nursing is responsible for hiring competent personnel and for the documentation of that competence. The department and individual nurse assume responsibility together for maintaining and documenting continuing maintenance of professional competence. The nursing service organization is responsible for the policies and procedures that internally govern practice and must strive to ensure that they reflect the current standard of care. Finally, the nursing organization is financially accountable for the use of personnel and resources that cause the employer to spend its money. The employer places faith in the nursing executive and nursing management to know the competency of its staff, to practice according to the standard of care, and to use personnel and resources for the maximum benefit of employer and patients.

Many nursing professionals have found themselves in situations that they considered unsafe because of staffing. Although it is the responsibility of nursing management to do its best to provide adequate staffing according to the acuity of the patient, the *individual* must assume responsibility for continuing to provide the best care possible under adverse conditions. Reporting perceived problems to nursing management, asking for help, and seeking assistance for resolution may be within the scope of the individual nurse, if handled correctly. Abandonment of the patient is never appropriate; nor is documentation of staffing issues in the patient's clinical record.

Risks to the Patients, Client, or Visitors

The nurse must keep in mind that the physician is charged with legal responsibility of diagnosis, treatment, and prescription. Because these responsibilities do not fall within the scope of nursing practice, it is vital that the nurse follow the prescribed policy and procedure for reporting perceived physician problems. Each institution is charged legally with having an established medical staff peer review system. The nurse should access this system through the risk management reporting system and the quality assessment/improvement department. Nursing should never be afraid to document concerns to the appropriate department while maintaining professional standards. The patient's medical record is *never* the correct vehicle to express concern or frustration regarding physician behavior or treatment of the patient. Remember, the nurse has the right to refuse to carry out any order that is believed to be in error or detrimental to the patient. The correct response to a physician who is demanding something the nurse in good conscience cannot perform is: "I cannot do that; however, I will let you speak to my supervisor." This tactic should be used all the way through the chain of nursing command.

The nursing administration bears the responsibility for defining nursing practice according to the acceptable standard of care. Caution must be used, however, in understanding the physician's request and in good nursing judgment regarding the urgent nature of the situation. Along this same line, the nurse, unless the situation is urgent, should not perform treatments or technical tasks for which she has not been educated. All nurses will eventually find themselves in situations for which their training or work experience has not prepared them.

Nurses share responsibility with many other health care providers for the general safety of the visitors who frequent the facility. Safety hazards such as spills, wet floors, and trip and fall hazards should be reported as soon as they are discovered, and anything that can be done to minimize the risk should be done.

Risks to the General Public

Nurses usually see their responsibility as falling within the scope of practice in the work environment, yet actions within the workplace and outside the health care facility may affect the general public. Recent publicity has been given to issues such as hazardous and infectious wastes that have been dumped into landfills. Homes and public buildings have been built on top of areas in which waste from health care institutions has been buried. Although, today, federal regulations govern the disposal of such substances by the health care provider, nurses play an integral role in maintaining compliance. It is as much the professional responsibility of the nurse to comply with disposal standards as it is to practice according to professionally set standards.

Not only do actions of a physical nature affect the general public, but also the demeanor and reputation of the professional nurse has a definite effect on how the public places trust in the health care provider. In the United States we have enjoyed the highest standard of health care ever known, yet we find the public suspicious and distrustful of the system and its providers. There are indeed occasions that have caused shame to the providers of health care; however, there are countless more occasions that spark faith and pride. At no other time has the profession of nursing had such opportunity to enhance its professional standing. Although federal and state mandates cause lower reimbursement and concerns among the public regarding access, the nursing profession is at the threshold of expanding that access and providing alternative forms of health care delivery. In some areas, nurses are already receiving *direct reimbursement for services.*

❖ JOINT COMMISSION ON ACCREDITATION OF HEALTH CARE ORGANIZATIONS

The JCAHO has recently recognized the importance of the risk management process to the quality of health care delivery. In response to that recognition, risk management was recognized with specific standards in 1990. Appropriately the JCAHO chose not to devote a specific chapter to the department of risk management but chose to weave the practice of risk management throughout all areas included in the survey. The standards in which risk management is cited include areas of highest risk such as medical staff credentialing and peer review, plant technology, and safety and nursing standards. Nursing must not only define the standards of practice but must have mechanisms in place to prove that the practice is indeed being carried out.

Within the realm of quality improvement the JCAHO has charged each department to design outcome indicators around high-risk, high-volume, and problem-prone areas of specific practice. The outcome indicators are included in both hospital and medical staff quality assessment programs. At the same time, JCAHO has directed that opportunities to improve care not only be identified but also that action plans and assessment of those plans result in improvement of the situation.

Quality improvement activities must be designed within the framework in which the individual department maintains control; however, the total quality improvement activity should lead to the identification of entire systems working within the health care organization that need improvement. The nursing service organization with the leadership of the nurse executive must remain open and willing to participate in the redesign of the system of providing health care that is identified with quality. As stated previously, nursing stands at the threshold of new and increased respect as a profession. Nursing has the responsibility to participate in the improvement of care delivery or the choice to hold back that improvement.

Within most health care organizations, nursing employs the largest group of professionals, uses the largest amount of resources, and has access to the highest numbers of patients. Nursing has the ability to promote or impede progress toward quality improvement. The quality improvement process embodies risk management principles in problem identification, the design of action plans to eliminate or reduce risk, and continuous assessment of effectiveness of actions.

❖ SAFETY/RISK MANAGEMENT IN QUALITY MANAGEMENT

Accidents produce economic and social loss. Productivity is impaired, as well as efficiency, and the standard of living is decreased. There are numerous aspects to consider when looking at accidents and accident prevention. There are moral and practical aspects that include the wasting of manpower and resources but also cause mental and physical suffering to the worker and his or her family. When a worker dies or is disabled because of work-related injuries, the economic consequences affect the worker, his or her family, the employer, and society. If the worker is partially or totally disabled, the cost of treatment and prolonged care or rehabilitation may be more than his or her annual income. The partially or totally disabled person may require public assistance and may be a drain on society. The society loses the products the worker would have produced, and there is a loss in taxes the worker would have generated. Those with permanent disability may have to be maintained the rest of their lives.

❖ EVOLUTION OF WORKMAN'S COMPENSATION PROGRAMS IN THE UNITED STATES

Before the nineteenth century there were no industrial systems in the United States. People worked on farms with very simple tools and no technology. No records of accidents were kept; therefore there were no recordings of injuries incurred. In the last half of the century the industrial process in America was in full swing, with companies rapidly expanding and production lines increasing. Although these systems were far superior in terms of production compared with the small craft shops of the past, they were far inferior in terms of the health and safety of the workers and the importance of the human element. Many of the deficiencies existed not because of a lack of concern but instead because of a lack of knowledge of the problems with health and safety that would be encountered by mass production. As mass production expanded, the accidents sharply increased and the general industrial health declined.

Finally, legislation was created to facilitate a safe work environment. The United States lagged far behind Europe in terms of the creation of workman's compensation programs. In 1867 the state of Massachusetts used factory safe inspectors and passed a state law that required factories that used dangerous machinery to have safeguards to prevent accidents and injuries. In 1893 legislators gained more insight into workman's compensation plans when John Graham Brock introduced his plan in Germany. Beginning in 1898 there was a trend to make employers financially liable for accidents on the job that resulted in injury to the employee. In 1902 the state of Maryland passed an Act for cooperative accident insurance, but it was of little benefit because the scope was narrow and the benefits were very poor. The benefits were paid only in the event of the death of the worker.

In 1908 President Theodore Roosevelt urged the passage of a workman's compensation act for federal employees. This was the first real workman's compensation plan in the United States. New York was the first state to adopt a workman's compensation law for the general public, but the coverage was limited to those workers whose jobs were considered hazardous.

Finally, the first effective workman's compensation plan was passed in Wisconsin, but it conflicted with the fourteenth amendment to the Constitution. In 1916 this went before the Supreme Court, and the Court ruled in favor of the plan. The major objective of the workman's compensation plan was to restore the earning power of the employee while recuperating and to aid the employee in returning to productive employment. Workman's compensation also provided an incentive for industries to reduce and prevent industrial accidents and the proper allocation of cost of the safety programs. Early in the twentieth century two major industrial powers in the United States initiated large organized safety programs, and other companies began to follow their lead by devising their own safety programs.

❖ SAFETY COUNCIL CREATION

The Association of Iron and Steel Electrical Workers initiated the first large-scale safety conference in 1911 in Milwaukee, and the following year the conference was called the National Council for Industrial Safety. Those in attendance agreed to meet the following year in New York. This safety conference later became the National Safety Council. The first conference was composed of a diverse group representing professionals, safety advisors, management leaders, and public officials, as well as representatives of the insurance industry.

❖ INDUSTRIAL SAFETY GROWTH AND RESULTS

The basis for all safety programs became the three Es of safety: *engineering, education,* and *enforcement.* Engineering was used to prevent accidents by designing safety mechanisms for machinery. Education and enforcement involved the education of the employees and the enforcement of established safety rules. This form of industrial safety based on the three Es was widely accepted between World War I and World War II. During World War II the country suffered a severe labor shortage and an even greater emphasis on the importance of industrial safety resulted. This great interest in safety did not lose momentum when the war came to an end.

There were dramatic results in reduced injury and accidents as the safety movement swept the nation. Since 1912 the death rates for persons in industry, age 25 to 64, have declined significantly. There has also been a radical decline in disabling injuries and thus savings to corporations. Since World War II there has been tremendous technologic advancement in industry; thus the safety issues have become more complex. Historically there has been an integrated approach to addressing safety issues with emphasis on environmental control, engineering, and the importance of the human component.

❖ NATIONAL SAFETY LEGISLATION ON THE CREATION OF OSHA

The first national safety legislation was not passed in the United States until 1970. The legislative piece was titled the Occupation Safety and Health Act (OSHA) and became effective April 28, 1971. This legislation affected every employer engaged in business. Regulations under OSHA encompassed the present with a look into the future and were comprehensive in nature. This legislation was a landmark piece. OSHA enforcement mechanisms included the Secretary of Labor, who is responsible for prosecution of violators, and the Occupational Safety and Health Review Commission was given the responsibility of adjudicating cases.

❖ OSHA FUNCTIONS AND REGIONAL PROGRAMS

The basic functions of OSHA included the following:
1. The development of safety and health standards and issue regulations
2. Provision for training programs for OSHA business employers and employees
3. Assistance in the establishment of federal agency programs to ensure effective compliance with regulations

OSHA regional programs are designed to provide support in the development of state compliance programs and attempt to ensure this compliance through state inspection programs and by offering technical assistance. The regional program also reviews and assesses the effectiveness and the efficiency of federal and state compliance as a system of checks and balances.

The administrative division collects data and designs information systems to facilitate the management of the OSHA programs. The National Institute for Occupational Safety and Health (NIOSH) was created under the provisions of OSHA, is charged with the responsibility for safety and health standards, and conducts research demonstrations related to occupational safety and health. NIOSH is also responsible for providing training programs for OSHA personnel.

❖ SAFETY IN HEALTH CARE

Florence Nightingale introduced basic sanitation such as open window ventilation for hospitals and the placement of fewer patients per ward. Semmelweis initiated routine handwashing as basic to the control of the spread of infectious disease. These early initiatives were designed for the protection of the patient but served the caretaker as well. Each attempt was a safety mechanism.

As medical technology advanced, there was recognition of new safety hazards for patients and caretakers. In the early 1900s when experimentation with x-ray was prevalent, many people were overexposed to radiation. The introduction of the first anesthetic gases posed the potential for injury by explosion.

Since this time there have been continual advances in technology and increased safety concerns and risks. In 1958 the American Hospital Association published a statement that emphasized the role of hospitals in setting the example to the public with respect to health education, preventive medicine, and job safety. This clearly gave new impetus for the safety movement.

In the early years health and safety programs were geared to the patient and not to the health care worker. Health care institutions were seen as safer places than other work environments. This belief was related to the idea that health professionals did not need assistance in maintaining their health and that a hospital was a place of treatment of disease rather than a place to maintain health. The easy access to the physician for health care workers made it easy to get informal consultation for health matters.

Safety and health in health care today encompass the patient, the facility staff, and visitors. Safety managers in the health care environment today must deal with safety issues and legal risks, as well as risks if there is a violation of applicable standards. Interestingly, law does not require health institutions to eliminate all hazards except those recognized by law. Safety officers must consider several issues when addressing safety hazards. He or she must determine which hazards are physically feasible to correct, those that are economically feasible to correct, and those that are not feasible to correct.

❖ JOINT COMMISSION SAFETY STANDARDS

The Joint Commission requires institutions to have safety programs to provide an environment that is free of hazards and to manage activities that reduce the risk of injury. A safety officer must be designated and assigned the responsibility for the development, implementation, and monitoring of the safety program. The safety program must include policies and procedures for safety in all departments and must be based on laws, regulations, and the experience of the institution. The safety program must be tailored to focus on those hazards that are related to the ages of the patients served and must have mechanisms for reporting hazards with identified resolutions. The Joint Commission requires the formation of a safety committee. The composition of the committee must minimally include a representative of administration in a facility and a representative from clerical and support services. There must be a specialized program in the facility to control and handle hazardous material and wastes such as chemotherapeutic agents and surgery suite waste.

❖ PSYCHOLOGIC FACTORS OF SAFETY/ELEMENT OF SAFETY ORGANIZATION

The effectiveness of the safety program hinges on the acceptance of the responsibility by the employees and can be achieved only by working with everyone. Psychologic factors related to the differences in people include motivation, emotions, general attitudes, and learning process and abilities.

The management in any organization must assume the responsibility for declaration of safety policies in a company. Management at all levels must be dedicated to the reduction of hazards and the promotion of a safe environment through education to all employees, and there must be a recording system for injuries, first aid applications, and periodic health examinations. Every facility must have an emergency preparedness plan, and buildings must meet life safety codes or the National Fire Protection Association's equivalent.

❖ SAFETY IN HEALTH CARE/NURSING

There are approximately 8 million health care workers in the United States, and hospitals employ approximately 4.5 million, with nurses representing the largest portion. Nurses play a key role in recognizing and addressing safety issues. Because nurses provide the majority of the patient care, their role is essential in recognizing and addressing risk issues. The continual technologic creations require the nurses to be educated and aware of the potential hazards.

From a clinical standpoint, safety encompasses a wide variety of potential hazards to the patient, such as medication administration, equipment usage, and appropriate isolation techniques. From a nurse's personal respect, care must be taken to utilize equipment properly—proper handwashing and disposal of waste—to prevent hazards for the nurses. Nurses must also be attuned to the environment and the potential hazards to other employees or visitors.

Each specialty area has hazards unique to the area. The reduction of hazards can be attributed to nursing knowledge and education of potential problems. Nurses must continually update their skills and develop a broad-based knowledge of safety measures. In a strong safety program, nursing must realize the critical role it plays in the safety and well-being of others and themselves.

The more technical the area, the greater the risks and potential risks. In areas such as critical care and surgery there are many pieces of equipment used in various combinations. In these areas, hazards include stray electrical current from the use of defibrillators and monitors. In surgery, safety issues may be related to exposure to radiation, the use of cautery, and the use of surgical instruments.

The proper functioning of equipment is a major safety concern, and nurses have a role to play in ensuring that equipment is functioning as expected. Preventive maintenance programs are an essential component of a safety program, involving not only patient care staff but also the maintenance department and technicians using the equipment.

Improper functioning of life-sustaining equipment such as respirators and blood circulation devices can not only make the difference in life or death but also affect the degree of recovery and the length of time it takes to rehabilitate. Diagnostic equipment poses a different type of concern related to proper diagnosis and treatment of disease and to the safety of those managing the equipment. Again, patient survival and length of recovery time are affected. Procedural techniques such as dressing changes and the disposal of hypodermic needles also pose a threat to patients and staff. The major key to safety is the reduction of hazards, the education of the staff, and the recognition by staff when equipment is malfunctioning. Reporting and repair are also essential.

Routine training programs can be beneficial in reducing safety hazards. Programs should be developed for new employees and when procedures are revised or new procedures introduced. Training programs are invaluable when large numbers of persons need the education or when overall performance is substandard. Key indicators of the need for an extensive training program are when more accidents or injuries occur at one facility compared with another of similar size and services and when there is a high labor turnover rate.

❖ SAFETY HAZARDS FOR HEALTH CARE WORKERS

As noted previously there are few workplaces as complex as the hospital or a health care environment. There are multitudes of hazards and potential hazards. Maintenance personnel are exposed to electrical hazards and solvents, and housekeepers are exposed to disinfectants and detergents. Food service personnel are subject to cuts and burns, and nurses are subject to infectious diseases and needle punctures. Radiology personnel are exposed to radiation, and the surgery personnel are exposed to burns, cuts, and puncture wounds.

❖ NURSING IMPLICATIONS/CLINICAL CONCERNS

Nurses play a principal role in the safety campaign in any facility. Because nurses provide the majority of the care to patients, they are often the first line in the defense of the patients' well-being. Proper nursing practice and following clinical procedures provide a safeguard for the patient and the nurse, as well as other facility staff.

Clinical safety concerns correlate to the health and safety of patients, visitors, and support staff. These concerns revolve around safe and optimal use of equipment and proper procedural techniques.

Administrative concerns are multiple, including legal, financial, reputation of the institution, ability to pass regulatory surveys, and staffing. Administration must support the safety program and encourage staff to adopt practices that are considered appropriate. Administrators must be educated and aware of the safety issues in a facility and be willing to support managers in the addressing of the issues. Strong administrative support of efforts to reduce hazards and promote a safe environment is critical.

❖ IMPLICATIONS FOR PRACTICE

Safety is integral in the risk management process and critical to the integrated quality management process. Risk management should have a close working relationship with safety in identifying potential risks and hazards. Quality assessment should work closely in identifying trends and noncompliance with recommendations.

The nurse is an important component in the safety portion of the risk management program. The integrated approach to quality improvement is not only the interaction between the functions (departments) of the quality improvement program, but also participation in all facets of the program is a part of the professional nurse's responsibility. Compliance with safety regulations, vigilance to safety hazards in the physical environment, and participation in the ongoing assessment of practice with the goal of identifying safety risks to patients, employees, and visitors should be a part of the routine performance of nursing responsibilities. Improved quality as an end result continues to enjoy much emphasis in health care. Attention to and performance of risk management and safety processes and responsibilities should result in the desired goal of improved quality.

❖ SUMMARY

Accidents produce economic and personal loss. Large industrial accidents led to the evolution of safety legislation to create a safe work environment. The accidents of the industrial revolution paved the way for the creation of safety as a field. Increased technologic advances focused attention on the complexities of health care delivery and the resultant risks and potential risks to patients and workers. OSHA laws and regulatory bodies such as JCAHO are essential, with risk of penalties and fines for noncompliance with standards. Administration, nursing, and all support staff play a critical role in the safety of the work environment and the reduction of hazards. Education and training are essential tools for hazard reduction and the promotion of safety by all managers. Risk management/safety is a vital component of an integrated quality management program. Open lines of communication between the other QM components are essential to the identification of potential risk issues and subsequent loss exposure.

REFERENCES

1. Asfal RC: *Industrial safety and health management,* New Jersey, 1984, Prentice-Hall.
2. Cazalas MW: *Nursing and the law,* Gaithersburg, Md, 1978, Aspen Systems.
3. Fiesta, J: *The law and liability, a guide for nurses,* New York, 1983, John Wiley & Sons.
4. Head GL, Horn S: *Essentials of the risk management process,* Malvern, Pa, 1985, Insurance Institute of America.
5. Hemelt MD, Mackert ME: *Dynamics of law in nursing and health care,* Reston, Va, 1978, Reston Publishing.
6. Joint Commission on Accreditation, *AMI,* Oakbrook, Ill, 1990.
7. *National Safety Council Manual,* 1988.
8. U.S. Department of Health & Human Services, Public Health Service, Centers for Disease Control, National Institute for Occupational Safety and Health, *Guidelines for protecting the safety and health of health care workers,* Sept. 1988.

CHAPTER

8

❖

Quality Management and Infection Control

❖ INTRODUCTION

Humanity has been plagued with infectious disease since the beginning of time. The first mention of the oldest known disease, rabies, was documented by Aristotle in a writing entitled *Historia Animalium* in 335 B.C. The epidemics affecting the Germans, Italians, and Spanish in 1173 are well documented. The Venetians coined the word *quarantine* in the fourteenth century in an effort to reduce infection by quarantining incoming ships for a specified period of time.

Ancient Egypt had well-developed methods of sewage disposal, and the Hebrews segregated lepers to avoid the spread of disease. During the Dark Ages community and personal health declined, but a resurgence of interest occurred during the Renaissance, the renewed era of scientific thought. By the nineteenth century the negative impact of poor health on social conditions and economic status was recognized, and in the 1830-1840s, the French developed the concept of medicine as a social and biologic science.

During the Industrial Revolution many people contracted fatal diarrheas, pneumonia, tuberculosis, measles, and smallpox. All of the diseases were linked to overcrowding, poverty, poor nutrition, poor sanitation, and lack of sewage disposal. There were no clean water systems; therefore water for all purposes was contaminated with industrial pollutants and human waste. Lack of knowledge and the lack of application of aseptic techniques contributed to the overwhelming number of patients who acquired wound infections after surgery. More than half of those patients died.

The first to theorize that infectious diseases were caused by a pathogenic microbe was Agostine Bossi, an Italian, in 1835. Pasteur published his writing on germ theory in 1878, and his work led to the scientific understanding of the connection between overcrowding and disease. Joseph Lister defined aseptic principles based on Pasteur's work and began to experiment with solutions to kill surgical wound bacteria.

Knowledge of the chemistry of bacteria and viruses led to techniques for treating water with chlorine and other chemicals strong enough to kill microbes but harmless to people. The discovery of sulfonamides in the early 1940s greatly reduced the number of deaths because of lung disease in the United States. Penicillin was successfully used on a British patient in 1941 and subsequently was used on the military in the United States and abroad during World War II.

The discovery and use of antibiotics during World War II improved the overall health of the military. From the end of the war until the mid-1960s federal funds were allocated to nurture and support medical research and education. Hospitals were built with legislative funding to improve health care access. The funding and research improved technology in diagnosis and treatment of disease. These innovations, although positive in terms of the availability of resources to treat and diagnose, also enhanced the risks for acquiring infections.

During this health care technology growth phase in the early 1950s, hospital infections were of little consequence because of the availability and widespread use of the sulfonamides and penicillin. In the late 1950s hospitals began to experience epidemics of staphylococcal infections that were becoming resistant to available antibiotics. By 1960 there was a pandemic of staph in both American and European hospitals. Striking increases in staph were noted in surgical wounds, newborn nurseries, and obstetric services. The seriousness of the problem was recognized by the hospitals, which began to develop internal infection control programs to deal with the problem. The early infection control programs consisted of patient review and clinical epidemiology with feedback to the hospital of infection rates. Lack of scientific evidence to validate the effectiveness of infection control methods hampered the success of many programs. Little evidence of the ability to reduce cost and a lack of administrative understanding and support also reduced the effectiveness of the early programs.

❖ NATIONAL RESPONSE TO STAPH PANDEMIC

The seriousness of the staph pandemic was recognized by a group of epidemiologists who decided to focus its attention on the problems faced by the hospitals. The major function of this group was to assist hospitals in developing effective strategies to deal with the pandemic. This group became known as the Centers for Disease Control (CDC). The American Hospital Association (AHA), working through its committee of infections, developed guidelines for hospitals and systems to control infections. The CDC and AHA began working together to address the issues. The collaboration resulted in the formulation of strategies for identifying causes for outbreaks of infections and used surveillance activities similar to those used in World War II for control of malaria. Recommendations for the early programs included the use of an epidemiologist for daily surveillance. Later revisions recommended the adoption of the British system of surveillance, using an infection control nurse to perform daily surveillance. The British system emphasized the observance of infection control practices and teaching staff appropriate infection control practices.

The infection control role in the United States was pioneered by Kay Wenzel, a nurse at Stanford, in 1963. Her primary functions were surveillance, supervision of isolation techniques, education of staff, and service as an advisor to the infection control committee.

In 1970 fewer than 10% of U.S. hospitals had formal infection control programs. By 1976 more than half of the hospitals had formal programs with written policies and procedures. No regulatory bodies monitored these programs or set standards, and JCAHO had only a general concept statement in its standards. Therefore hospitals were responding to an increased awareness of the problem of infections and were attempting to address the problems.

❖ EPIDEMIOLOGY

Epidemiology can be defined as the study of factors that contribute to the incidence, distribution, and control of disease, defect, disability, and death. Historically epidemiology focused on understanding and control of epidemic diseases. Epidemiology now focuses on control of health problems and applies epidemiologic techniques to health problems, as well as communicable diseases.

Theories regarding the cause of illness have evolved over time. During what is described as the "religious era," disease was believed to be the result of divine intervention as punishment for misdeeds. Following this period, disease was believed to be caused by various physical forces such as harmful mists or miasmas. The bacteriologic era began with the discovery of specific organisms as the reason for specific diseases. From 1850 to 1880 disease was believed to be due to uncleanliness. From 1880 to 1920 the emphasis on disease control was based on bacteriology. The health promotion phase occurred from 1920 to 1960, and even until the present, emphasis on health as a right has increased technology and accessibility.

Because initial epidemiology focused on acute communicable disease, as the incidence of communicable disease declined, epidemiologists began to concentrate on chronic diseases. The ultimate concern for epidemiology is prevention of disease and maintenance of health.

❖ THE SCIENTIFIC BASIS FOR INFECTION CONTROL

In the early 1970s the CDC began to question whether surveillance and the recommended control measures were indeed effective. Concern was growing that no scientific data substantiated the methods of infection control endorsed by the AHA and CDC were effective. Many feared that, with cost reductions and lack of validation of techniques, hospitals would begin to shut down infection control programs.

In January 1974 the CDC began an extensive three-phase study on infection control in hospitals, which was called the Senic Study on the Efficacy of Nosocomial Infection Control (see box). Phase I was designed to calculate measures of surveillance and control activities. Phase II encompassed on-site assessments of sample hospitals where detailed descriptions were given of the ongoing infection control program. Phase III was a medical records survey. All data were collected by 1984, computerized, and edited for accuracy.

Senic Project Phases

Phase I	Calculation of measures of surveillance and control activities
Phase II	On-site assessment of sample hospitals with detailed descriptions of ongoing infection control programs
Phase III	Medical records survey

Data revealed a 32% reduction in nosocomials in facilities in which a four-component infection control program existed. The four critical elements of the programs were surveillance, intensive control, an adequately trained infection control coordinator, and a trained infection control staff.

❖ NOSOCOMIAL INFECTION RATES AND TYPES

Nosocomial infections are those that occur during the hospitalization but are neither present nor incubating at the time of admission. Since the staph pandemics of the 1960s and the invention of infection control programs, data indicate that surgical wound infections account for one fourth of all nosocomials. Many variables affect surgical wound infection rates. As mentioned previously, as technology increases, infection rates also increase. A greater potential exists for adverse outcomes when more sophisticated and technical techniques and equipment are used. Patients who have multiple chronic diseases live longer. Those patients are frequently elderly, their conditions are more compromised, they are therefore more susceptible to infection. A certain level of bacteria is ever present, and simply making an incision increases the odds for an infection. Surgical technique is also a factor in nosocomials. Increased technology in surgical instrumentation creates one possibility, and the use of that equipment poses another threat. Increased technology and perfection of surgical techniques often mean greater lengths of time involved in the performance of the procedure, as well as more persons in and around the surgical suite, which increases the potential for a wound infection.

Forty percent of all nosocomials are related to urinary tract infections, which are a result of catheter use, and many last for extended periods of time. Many patients are required to perform self-catheterization and have difficulty or must rely on a caretaker to perform the procedure. Pneumonia accounts for 19% of nosocomials, and bloodstream infections account for 5% of nosocomials.

The original CDC pilot study of 1970 revealed an average nosocomial rate of 5%. By the mid-1980s, this rate was expected to be at 7%. The anticipated increase was projected based on increased technology. Larger hospitals had more nosocomials than did smaller hospitals, and hospitals with higher surgical case loads had more nosocomials, regardless of size. The magnitude of the nosocomial problem was directly related to the degree of underlying risk of patients. The average surveillance activities detect only about one half of the nosocomials, and the most intensive surveillance efforts detect only three fourths of the infections. The cost of nosocomials to the institution is measured by added days hospitalized or added length of stay, increased hospital costs, and decreased revenues. Patient mortality related to nosocomial infection is approximately 10%.

❖ SURVEILLANCE BY OBJECTIVES

Surveillance by objectives (SBO) has been recognized by the CDC as an effective means of surveillance. Different surveillance systems are designed to monitor and control various types of infections. Annual prevention outcomes are written by infection control staff, and objectives are written. Education of professional and medical staff is a major component in the overall program.

❖ JCAHO AND INFECTION CONTROL

When the staph pandemic occurred in the early 1960s, the Centers for Disease Control organized and began to assist hospitals in establishing infection control programs. The AHA joined the CDC effort, and they worked together to assist hospitals in establishing programs to reduce infections and improve quality of care. Before 1976 there was no federal pressure to establish infection control programs although most hospitals were already doing so. Since that time the Joint Commission has developed and refined standards to reflect the CDC and AHA guidelines. Hospitals are now required by JCAHO to have hospital-wide infection control programs that include surveillance. The programs are required to have written policies and procedures that describe types of surveillance, systems to collect and analyze data, and activities in every department to prevent and control infections. JCAHO requires specific policies for decontamination and sterilization activities and that a multidisciplinary committee meet at least once a quarter to discuss infection control problems, actions, and follow-up.

Today emphasis on control and prevention is increased, and programs are allowed more latitude in surveillance activities. Surveillance types include any occurrence of community acquired or nosocomial infections because of unusual pathogens, epidemics, unusual clusters, and any nosocomial exceeding a baseline level. Pertinent findings are reported to the multidisciplinary committee for follow-up action.

❖ FUTURE IMPLICATIONS/BENEFITS

Continued development of technology in the treatment and diagnosis of illness will increase the potential for infections. The fact that many patients are elderly, with chronic illnesses, predisposes a large percentage of the population to infectious diseases. Nosocomial infections are emerging as a major health problem, and some studies suggest that nosocomial infections are the tenth leading cause of death in the United States. Health care entities are challenged to provide an array of services while ensuring the quality of care and controlling costs.

Effective infection control programs will continue to positively affect the financial viability by decreased lengths of stay and resource use. Favorable survey results can enhance marketing strategies and encourage the use of other services provided. Most important, effective programs decrease mortality, increase productivity of the individual, and serve as a benefit to society.

As technology increases and health care delivery diversifies, the need for sophisticated infection control programs will also increase. Strong administrative support will continue to be crucial to a successful program.

❖ INFECTION CONTROL AND CONTINUOUS QUALITY IMPROVEMENT

The Senic project results indicated a significant reduction in nosocomial infections in facilities with a four-component infection control program. The components of surveillance, control efforts, a trained coordinator, and staff are no less important when CQI is embraced. Funding and specification of problem areas will be necessary, but the manner in which the information is handled will be different. Under CQI, improving quality through the infection control program will involve enhanced training, technical innovation, and procedural improvements, as opposed to punishing individuals. Improved quality under CQI will rely on defining process failures while integrating traditional infection control components.

❖ INFECTION CONTROL ADMINISTRATIVE CONCERNS

The CEO or administrative support will be vital to successful programs. Administration's awareness of the approaches to infection control that are successful will be helpful in soliciting physician and professional staff support. The success of the programs can be measured by decreased malpractice claims, lengths of stay, and resource use. Prospective pricing adds another impetus to funding and supporting infection control programs that improve quality and decrease cost.

❖ INFECTION CONTROL AND NURSING

Nursing process and epidemiologic processes are very similar. *Nursing process* involves the use of assessing, planning, implementing, and nursing research. *Epidemiology process* includes identifying the problem, determining the extent of the problem, planning a strategy, implementing the control program, and evaluating the research.

As primary care givers, nurses play a pivotal role in disease prevention, intervention, and recognition. In the four major categories of nosocomials, nurses play an important role in prevention and recognition. Surgical wounds can be contaminated by poor technique during surgery or after surgery. Nurses may observe poor technique and may recognize signs of infection very early. Bloodstream infections can result from contamination during intravenous catheter insertion or poor care after insertion, and nursing can affect both. Pneumonias and lung complications can result from poor postoperative care or poor or inadequate preoperative teaching. Nurses play the major role in teaching and aftercare. Urinary tract infections are often the result of faulty sterile technique or lack of care after insertion. Again nursing has the ability to affect this care.

Sicker patients and increased technology dictate the need for nurses to continue to monitor their own practices and those of their peers. Nurses must continue to gain knowledge and update skills to meet the changing needs. Nursing can serve as a resource to the infection control program and can alert physicians to the earlier indication of an infection. Nurses can set the example for peers and other professional staff and can educate the patient and family members as to the appropriate practices.

❖ INFECTION CONTROL IN LONG-TERM CARE

Long-term care units provide a variety of levels of care to a larger group of the population today. The introduction of DRGs and PPS has caused patients to be discharged from the acute care setting much earlier than in previous years. Many of these patients require interim care in a long-term care facility, patients in long-term care units often require higher levels of care and more compromise than their predecessors. Long-term care units provide a variety of infection control challenges in today's environment. Some long-term care units provide care in semiprivate or ward settings, thus increasing the odds for cross-contamination. Urinary and bowel incontinence is also a major problem in some long-term care units, which in itself creates a challenge for control of infections. Outbreaks of infectious disease, as in acute care, can result in increased lengths of stay, increased morbidity and mortality, resource consumption with subsequent increased cost, and readmission to acute care facilities.

❖ INFECTION CONTROL IN HOME HEALTH CARE

The effects of PPS and DRG inception have also promoted the use of home health care as a means of receiving health care outside the acute care arena. New approaches to care of the dying have also played a role in diverting patients toward having care in the home. As in long-term care, home health care patients are often sicker, more debilitated, and require high level care with invasive technology. In this setting, patients, home health care staff, and families are at risk for developing infection; therefore infection control in the home is also critical. Generally infection rates for home health care patients are lower than those in acute or long-term care units, but basic infection control principles are still very important and must be adapted.

Factors that affect in-home infections are availability of resources including human resources, intelligence of care giver(s), and the ability to teach. Isolation techniques are a little more difficult to handle in the home, and waste disposal of dressings, syringes, and other items are of great concern. Simple handwashing may pose a problem if running water and soap are inaccessible. Disinfection of the home is more difficult to accomplish but can be done. Equipment used by the home health care staff and taken in and out of the home must be kept free of contaminants; otherwise, it would create the potential for cross-contamination of other home health care patients. Reporting of infection rates to the central department for home health care is more difficult because many agencies are not hospital based, nor are all patients referred from one source. Home health care agencies should keep their own programs and records and must recognize that infections detected after the first 48 hours after a hospital discharge should be considered nosocomial. Other infections may require reporting to local and state health agencies, according to state laws.

❖ SUMMARY

Humanity has always been plagued with disease and has made many attempts to control disease entities. The discovery of antibiotics improved the health of the general population but may have led to some complacency regarding spread of infections. In the 1960s infection control programs emerged in hospitals under the guidance of the CDC and AHA to deal with worldwide staph pandemics that were occurring. Guidelines were developed and proved effective with the Senic project, which are reviewed and revised as indicated. Nosocomial, or hospital acquired, infections continue to pose a problem as technology improves. The cost in pain and suffering because of nosocomials is immeasurable but definitely increases patient care cost, resource utilization, and mortality rates. Patients in home health care and long-term care require higher levels of care than their predecessors. Infection control in long-term care and home health care poses many challenges, particularly in the home in which the environment and resource availability are less controlled.

Infection control programs will remain important as levels of health care and settings shift and technology increases. The public and governmental demand for quality will continue to place demands on institutions for effective prevention and infection control programs.

REFERENCES

1. Bennett JV: Human infections: economic implications and prevention, *Ann Intern Med.*II. 89:5, 1978.
2. Brown J: *The 1990 quality assurance professionals study guide,* 1990, Managed Care Consultants.
3. Burgess W, Ragland EC: *Community health nursing: philosophy, process, practice,* Norwalk, Conn., 1983, Appleton-Century-Crofts.
4. Chase, A: *The biological imperatives,* New York, 1971, Holt, Rinehart & Winston.
5. Clark MJD : *Community nursing, health care for today and tomorrow,*Reston, 1984, Reston Publishing.
6. Haley R: Managing hospital infection control: a strategy for reducing complications, *American Hospital Association Manual,* Oct. 1985, American Hospital Publishing.
7. Kritchevsky S, Simmons B: Continuous quality improvement, concepts & applications for physician care, *JAMA* p 362, Oct. 2, 1991.
8. Simmons B, Trusler M, Roccaforte J, Smith P, Scott R: Infection control for home health, *Infect Control Hosp Epidemio* 11:362, 1990.
9. *Tennessee Peer Review Organization Manual,* April 1, 1989.
10. Wenzel KS: The role of the infection control nurse, *Nurs Clin North Am* 5:89, 1970.

CHAPTER

9

Integration of Quality Management Processes

❖ INTEGRATION: BY DEFINITION

INTEGRATION is a popular word in health care today. Departments are integrated, meaning that they are combined for better use of existing personnel. Often the consequence is that staff members are asked to do more with the same number of positions or full-time equivalents (FTEs). Another result may be the elimination of positions as remaining staff members are expected to learn new roles in combination with the previous ones. Because this process is not always well accepted and may be thought of as threatening, the term *integration* is not always viewed as a positive concept.

The word *integration* has several meanings and inferences. The *New Webster's Medical Dictionary* describes integration as ". . . constituting a whole; assimilation . . ."[12] To *assimilate* means ". . . to make similar to . . . to take up and make part of itself or oneself . . . to absorb . . . to digest . . . incorporate . . . to become alike . . ."[14] It is no wonder the use of this word is not always well received. Most people do not want to be "absorbed" or "digested" so that everyone is "alike." This definition explains why there may be resistance to the process of integration.

Other definitions must be explored to clarify the concept. To *integrate* means ". . . to make whole or complete by adding or bringing parts together . . . to unify . . . to remove barriers . . . to organize various traits into one harmonious personality."[14] This is a more positive approach and one that must be used when describing the unification of the various processes of quality management.

❖ INTEGRATION AND THE QUALITY MANAGEMENT PROCESS

To integrate the quality management processes, the commonalities must be defined. Segregation of the components must end as each area is brought into equal membership in the mutual goal: a defined, proactive plan to provide quality patient care in any setting where nursing is practiced. Integrated quality management is mandatory as outcome monitoring becomes a reality in the health care industry. Through integrated quality management, positive patient care outcomes can be achieved, documented, and measured.

All areas of quality management relate to each other. Often there is an overlap of processes. In quality assessment there is monitoring and evaluation of outcomes documented in the medical record as there is in utilization management, infection control, and risk and safety management. The chart remains the key document for these activities because it is the only total record of the treatments and care provided to the patient.

Data collection for aggregation, analysis, and trending is necessary for quality assessment, utilization management, infection control, and risk and safety management. To analyze any current problems in the various areas of quality management, data must be collected from records, incident reports, quality assessment studies, utilization management reports, and infection control surveillance records. Other data sources include interviews with patients, patient satisfaction surveys, and observation of the care provided. This same data must be analyzed and trended so that an appropriate action plan can be developed. Any key part that is missing will result in a less than optimal quality plan for the patient receiving health care in any setting. This would be similar to trying to see the total picture with missing puzzle pieces.

The challenge to integrate quality management is to produce useful data and analysis of opportunities for improvement. Often health care facilities find themselves data "rich" but information "poor." Data provided to managers without adequate interpretation is both useless and frustrating for the manager. The challenge is to provide integrated quality information that is useful, manageable, and comprehensive.

The processes of integrated quality management face the same obstacles common to health care, with limited resources in staff, time, and automation. Although everyone is interested in providing quality patient care, the integrated processes of quality assessment and improvement, utilization management, risk and safety management, and infection control demand accountability and responsibility in an already pressured environment.

Quality management may be thought of as crossing too many lines of authority and threatening to both administrators and professional practitioners. This resistance may further produce fragmentation in the planning of quality patient care.

❖ THE INTEGRATED QUALITY MANAGEMENT MODEL

Nurses must be involved on a daily basis in determining the professional aspects of their practice that are appropriate for monitoring and evaluation. Nurses should write down indicators and collect and analyze data. Then they can put their findings into practice to improve patient care outcomes.

Nurses are key players in total organizational quality management. The nurses of most agencies provide the bulk of the health care services delivered. It is important that they be active participants in quality improvement teams, not only on their units but also in the total organization. Nurses can learn to use the tools needed to improve care, such as flow charts, paretos, and "fishbone" cause-and-effect diagrams. It is appropriate that nurses participate actively because they are the most available and consistent professionals in the patient's care in most settings.

Neuman's System Model: A Conceptual Framework

The integrated quality management concept can be explained through use of Neuman's Systems Model. Neuman states that her model provides a process by which nurses can approach varied practice problems and understand the patient and the environment. She describes a nurse's role as being concerned with the variables that stress the patient. The nurse in Neuman's model is the "actor" or intervener whose role is to minimize the patient's exposure to stressors or at least minimize the effects of those stressors. Once the problem has been identified, the nurse must make a decision regarding the priority of the planned intervention.[11]

Neuman furthers defines the goal of nursing[10]:

> ... to assist individuals, families, and groups to attain and maintain a maximum level of total wellness by purposeful interventions ... aimed at reduction of stress factors and adverse conditions which either affect or could effect optimal functioning in a given client situation.

In summary, by using this model the nurse can address (1) the patient as being in various states of health, (2) the environment as both internal and

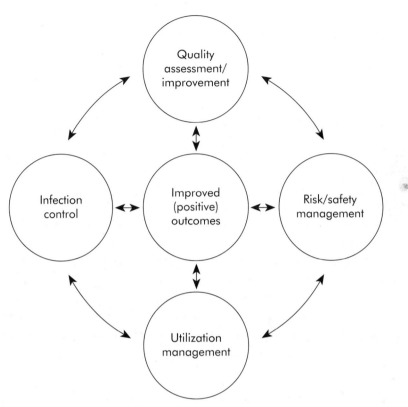

FIGURE 9-1
Integrated quality management model: improved (positive) outcomes.

external to the patient and in a state of flux (with stressors), and (3) the nurse as the intervener in the total process.[4]

Nurses can approach varied practice problems by using the Neuman model. The nurse has a goal to intervene in patient care to effect a positive outcome. Through integrated quality management the nurse minimizes the stressors in the health care environment through quality assessment and improvement, risk and safety management, utilization management, and infection control. If the stress has already occurred, the nurse assesses the adverse outcome to lessen its effects. The quality management process can then be improved to prevent adverse outcomes in the future.

This model can be depicted as in Fig. 9-1. Improved quality (positive) outcomes can occur in patient care and are the center of the integrated quality management system. The processes of quality assessment, risk/

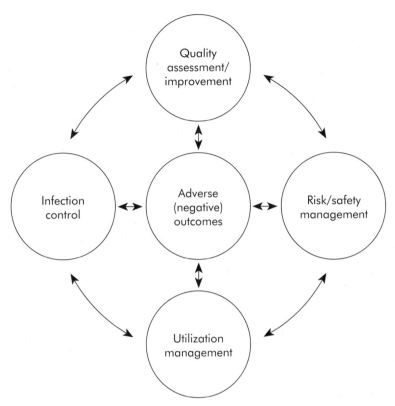

FIGURE 9-2
Integrated quality management model: adverse (negative) outcomes.

safety management, infection control, and utilization management form circles around this "center." Quality assessment provides the scope of care, and then each remaining process adds additional "stressor" evaluation opportunities. The total process is integrated to produce improved positive outcomes. The center can also be adverse (negative) patient care outcomes (Fig. 9-2). The same evaluation process occurs to assess the implications for integrated quality management.

Quality Management Tool: Cause-and-Effect Diagram

A quality management tool that is most helpful in evaluation of the integrated quality management processes is the cause-and-effect diagram, known as the fishbone diagram because of its shape. The originator was Dr.

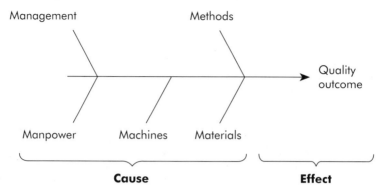

FIGURE 9-3
Cause-and-effect diagram.

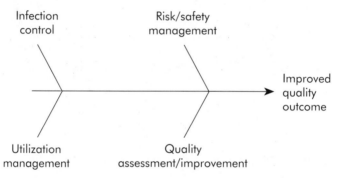

FIGURE 9-4
Integrated quality management cause-and-effect diagram.

Ishikawa.[6] The diagram is used most effectively in brainstorming discussions to define all possible factors that influence a situation. The *effect* can be either a desirable or undesirable condition, event, or situation that is the end result of a system of *causes*. The fishbone diagram often has as its *causes* four or five categories. These can include manpower, materials, methods, machines, and management. Fig. 9-3 demonstrates this process.[2]

To improve patient care, staff members can adapt this cause-and-effect diagram for use with integrated quality management. The nurse manager and staff would brainstorm the causes of an adverse patient care outcome, based on the processes of integrated quality management. Fig. 9-4 demon-

CHAPTER 9 INTEGRATION OF QUALITY MANAGEMENT PROCESSES 127

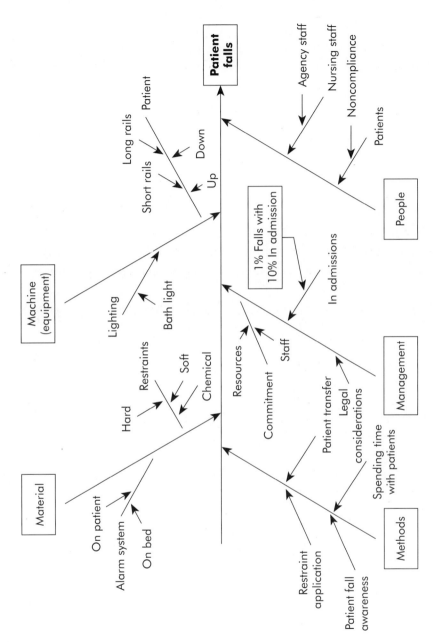

FIGURE 9-5
Cause-and-effect diagram; patient falls. (From Bush D: *Quality management through statistics . . . the next quality assurance generation*, Blackwood NJ, 1990, Diversified Business Associates—Health Education Division, p. 237.)

strates this model. The possible causes would then be prioritized by high risk, high volume, and problem prone (quality assessment), and another cause-and-effect diagram would be drawn for each quality management process that created an adverse outcome (Fig. 9-5.) This provides further analysis of specific problems in processes of care delivery. Through trending and analysis of these specific processes, a proactive monitoring and evaluation process can be implemented proactively.

To make a cause-and-effect diagram, the nurses must first determine the quality characteristic that is named at the point of the arrow. Second, the group brainstorms and writes down the main factors causing the quality characteristic. Each of these forms a "branch." Finally, on each branch, the group writes down more detailed factors related to the "branch" cause, making "twigs." On each of these, further causal definition can be made.[2]

There are many benefits to the nurse when using this diagram. Ishikawa defines these as the following[6]:

1. The creation process itself is educational. It gets a discussion going, and people learn from each other.
2. It helps a group focus on the issue at hand, reducing complaints and irrelevant discussions.
3. It results in an active search for the cause.
4. Data often must be collected.
5. It demonstrates the level of understanding. The more complex the diagram, the more sophisticated the workers are about the process.
6. It can be used for any problem.

The appendix includes case studies that use this model with a cause-and-effect diagram to demonstrate the application of integrated quality management.

❖ STRATEGIES FOR INTEGRATING QUALITY MANAGEMENT PROCESSES

Many practitioners are more knowledgeable about one process of integrated quality management than the others. Perhaps one nurse has had previous experience in quality assurance (assessment) and values the excellent results of problem identification and solutions for improving patient care delivery. Another likes risk management and can readily point out the risks that affect patient care. Some nurses appear "naturals" in infection control. Still others enjoy the challenge of identifying areas in which resources are wasted, and improvement translates into better patient care and use of staff as in utilization management.

Several strategies can be implemented to clarify the misconception that the nurse must "be all things to all people" in integrated quality management. Nurses must learn to value the quality management department of the hospital as a collaborative resource but not responsible for the quality of care provided at the unit level. Indeed these professionals are invaluable as guides in quality management and perhaps can provide some assistance in education, quality management implementation, and data collection and analysis. However, the accountability for quality management in any nursing practice setting rests with each level of nursing from manager to staff.

Quality management must be incorporated into nursing education at all levels. Early in the student nurse's career, recognition of the processes of integrated quality management and the implications for patient care must be emphasized. Educators themselves must learn the value of quality management and become mentors for nursing students. Care plans must address quality and include all processes of integrated quality management to produce positive patient care outcomes.

In graduate education the clinical nurse specialist and nurse administrator must recognize the impact of quality management on advanced nursing practice. In the leadership standards of the JCAHO *Agenda for Change*, advanced practice nurses are held accountable for assessing and planning for quality patient care. Advanced practice nurses are in the position to provide leadership and mentoring to the other nurses in the various practice settings. The quality management concept must be taught and practiced in graduate nursing schools, not as an elective but integrated into the core curriculum as a horizontal thread. In this way students will build on their knowledge base with each new clinical and course. Quality management must be a major consideration in all areas of advanced nursing practice.

Another strategy for integrating quality management into nursing practice is to discuss both the fears and the positive outcomes of the process with the nurse manager and staff. Integration does not mean total proficiency in quality assessment, utilization management, infection control, and risk and safety management. It does require a total commitment to learning to integrate the total concept into the daily activities of nursing practice. It also demands a knowledge base that can be developed by reading current literature, participating in committees that address the various quality processes, and attending workshops on the processes of quality management. A willingness to rethink the current approach to practice is necessary, with quality management always in the forethought. The fear that everyone must know everything or that there is an individual at fault when an adverse outcome occurs must be dispelled. This is a learning process and a change in the paradigm of previous education and experience. The positive results are better patient care outcomes and empowerment of the nursing profession.

Quality management should be a part of each nurse's orientation, which is the best time to express the expectation of participation in quality management as a management philosophy. Addressing quality management activities in the nurse's performance appraisal will both emphasize its importance and allow recognition for nurses who actively participate. Scheduling inservice time for each nurse to present a case study of quality management patient care planning will help the presenting nurse, as well as the attending nurse at the inservice.

Nurses who successfully integrate quality management into the various practice settings should be encouraged to publish articles describing their experience in facility newsletters, as well as in nursing journals. So often the published articles on quality management are found in trade journals specifically read by quality management professionals, such as quality assessment journals. It is important that descriptions of unit-based integrated quality management processes be published in journals read by the practicing nurse, such as clinical or administrative journals. This is another strategy for supporting the integrated quality management concept.

Nurses can also present their experience with integrated quality management at conferences and workshops. Both clinical and administrative conferences welcome abstracts on integrated quality management. This should be encouraged by the enlightened nursing administrator.

Issues and responsibilities that occur with implementing unit-based quality management must be recognized and addressed. Because the departments currently assigned to perform the individual processes may feel threatened by nursing integrating quality management into practice, nursing managers should ask for their assistance in implementing integrated quality management at the unit level. Traditionally the departments of quality assurance (assessment), utilization management, infection control, and safety and risk management have had sole responsibility for these processes. There may be some fear of lost identity.

These departments may feel diminished authority and influence as nursing integrates the quality management process into daily patient care practice. The nursing manager and staff must be sensitive to that and include these departments as the authorities that they are: they have knowledge and experience that is valuable to implementing quality management at the unit level. Invite them to meetings and ask them to join unit-based quality management committees. Remember, this is no time to reinvent the wheel. Wasting available resources is poor utilization management.

❖ EXAMPLES OF INTEGRATED QUALITY MANAGEMENT IN VARIOUS PRACTICE SETTINGS

Examples of integrated quality management can be used to demonstrate the implementation process of this concept in nursing practice in various settings. Examples of implementation in an acute care setting, long-term care setting, home health care setting, and outpatient setting follow.

Acute Care: Integrated Quality Management

Diabetes mellitus is a complex disease that accounts for more than $14 billion in health care costs annually. Twenty-four million hospital days are attributed to diabetes treatment per year, with hospitalization more likely in 2.4 times as many people as other diseases. The length of stay in the hospital is 2 to 3 days longer than the nondiabetic patient.[3]

Quality assessment and improvement are an important part of managing the diabetic in the acute care setting, which presents a challenge as new technology and procedures are introduced. One example is glucose monitoring with high technology equipment. Not only must staff be proficient in using the technology but also the meter and strips used must be accurate because treatment is based on the readings from the high-tech machines. Daily controls must be monitored, as well as follow-up documented on problematic patients.[1]

A risk management concern in this scenario would be the competency of the staff to perform such a high-tech procedure with critical implications for the patient's treatment. Documentation of an educational program that included training, review of policies and procedures, performing and documenting the process, and steps to take if the equipment is faulty would be necessary. Subsequent credentialing would be necessary to maintain competency in this procedure. Credentialing is a shared responsibility, based on quality assessment and risk management concerns.

Utilization management assessment would include monitoring the documented need for continued stay in the acute care setting, based on the severity of illness and intensity of service needed by the diabetic patient. A question the nurse might ask in the utilization side of quality management is: "Were glucose monitoring tests performed in a timely manner so that no delay in treatment resulted in increased hospital length of stay?" Another appropriate question would be: "Has teaching for home monitoring been initiated to allow safe transfer for the diabetic patient to another level of care such as home care?"

Another common problem for diabetics is infection. The infection control part of integrated quality management would examine any unsafe exposure to pathogens that decreased the patient positive outcome through infectious illness at the hospital. Any infection contracted at the hospital would result in an extended hospital stay, a utilization management concern. Likewise, any extended stay in the hospital increases the diabetic patient's chances of contracting another infection.

As demonstrated by this scenario, the diabetic patient is a common acute care patient whose patient care outcomes can be influenced by the implementation of integrated quality management in nursing practice. In this way nurses can affect the quality of care received by the diabetic patient in the acute care setting.

Long-Term Care: Integrated Quality Management

There are more aging Americans than ever before. In fact the adult of 85 years and older is the fastest growing part of the 65 and older population.[8] With aging comes chronic illness and functional disabilities that require some form of long-term care. Some estimate that as many as 5 million elderly require some degree of long-term care in the United States today.[8] Long-term care can include institutional care or home or community care.

The Omnibus Budget Reconciliation Act of 1987 (OBRA 87) requires that long-term care facilities have quality assurance (assessment) programs.[5] OBRA mandates a minimum data set be assessed on patient admission and at regular intervals, with emphasis of the survey process on outcome data. An example of a nursing outcome indicator is: "The resident shall be dressed in clean clothes, hair combed, nails trimmed/clean, face shaven, and be well-groomed overall each day." In addition, standards must address vision and hearing needs; activities of daily living; fluid and nutrition intake; cognitive, behavioral, and social functioning; and prevention and care of pressure sores. Regulations require an annual quality assessment and assurance plan.

Risk management is another important part of quality management in long-term care. There are standards that address the use of drugs and potential for accidents. Falls are a chief problem among the elderly, and a fall prevention program is important to quality management in the older adult. There are also standards that address the use of physical and chemical restraints. Many of these vary with the degree of physical and mental dependence that dictates a long-term care nursing status. Quality assessment monitors are built around these patient needs also to evaluate any problems in maintaining the standards.

OBRA also addressed the appropriateness and necessity of health care provided by individual departments or individuals. This is where utilization management, or utilization of resources, is noted. Different degrees of resident dependence require a varying level of staffing. Some residents are self-sufficient, and others must be fed and bathed. Assessing the appropriate level of resources needed is not only a part of utilization management but also is part of risk management as well. If the level of care needed is not appropriately assessed and the patient has an adverse outcome such as a fall or a burn, quality care is not achieved.

Infection control is paramount as the residents live day to day in the same, close environment. One of the OBRA standards for assessing quality of care provided by institutions addresses the use of urinary catheters. This is because urinary catheters can be a primary cause of urinary tract infections. The regulations ensure that the catheter is needed; thus the risk of infection is necessary, rather than that the catheter is for staff convenience. Again an appropriate nursing outcome monitor would be to study the patients who required catheterization and who received an adverse outcome—a urinary tract infection. This is also a good utilization study as the appropriateness of the patient for the treatment with a urinary catheter would be questioned.

Institutional long-term care offers many opportunities for integrated quality management. Certain nursing assessments and interventions can produce positive outcomes in the long-term care patient. In long-term care, nursing quality management can make a difference in the quality of life for the patient.

Home Care: Integrated Quality Management

Home care continues to grow as a setting for providing health care. It is estimated that by the year 2000, 70% of the nation's health care services will be provided outside the hospital.[9] The challenge to every home care provider is to provide quality care in the home that results in positive patient care outcomes.

Home infusion therapy is a service that is growing in utilization. The current home infusion therapy market has increased 30% for the past 3 years, with continued projected growth of 20% to 25%.[7] Currently many intravenous therapies are provided in the home, such as antibiotic therapy, pain management, prelabor management, and parenteral nutrition. A quality assessment process would identify home infusion therapy as a scope of service provided by the agency. An important aspect of care would be intravenous medication administration. A quality outcome indicator might be intravenous site drainage, which indicates infection, or phlebitis. Thus quality assessment and infection control are integrated.

Risk management is of utmost importance for the home infusion therapy patient. At home there is less control of the patient's care. The family is taught to monitor the intravenous site for signs of infection and inflammation between nurse visits. A major risk management concern is whether the patient and/or family were taught to care for the site before hospital discharge. Another risk management concern is whether the care giver is capable of providing the care necessary for the patient. Is the home environment safe for this kind of high-tech therapy? What are the risks or dangers in the home? Are the home care nurses credentialed to provide infusion services safely?

Utilization management questions the appropriateness of treatment in infusion therapy in the home. Is this the appropriate level of care for this patient? Again, are the resources in the home adequate for infusion therapy? Is there reimbursement for this therapy? Could this treatment be given effectively through another route such as by mouth or injection, or was this the only alternative?

Infection control, though difficult in the hospital, is even harder to manage in the home. The infusion therapy patient returns to his own environment. The family is taught to change the dressing over the intravenous insertion site, using sterile technique. No one watches, as in the hospital. No one is down the hall to call, as in the hospital. If the site is contaminated, the patient risks an additional infection and possible extension of his therapy affecting utilization management. Monitoring secondary infections is an appropriate outcome indicator for quality assessment and infection control on the home infusion patient.

As home care increases as an alternative to hospitalization, especially with the advent of high-tech therapies, integrated quality management is a necessary part of any home care program. Nursing practice in the home is a natural setting to practice quality management. With less control of the environment, good documentation of quality assessment will empower and protect the professional home care nurse.

Outpatient Surgery: Integrated Quality Management

Another popular patient care setting is the outpatient surgery area. Many surgeries such as hernia repair, tubal laparoscopic examinations, plastic surgeries, and cataract operations that once required hospitalization are performed in the outpatient setting. In fact almost 50% of all surgery is now performed on an outpatient basis.[9] Indeed the nurse practicing in the outpatient surgery setting has a unique challenge: to complete the nursing process and provide quality patient care for the few hours the patient is in the outpatient setting. This must be done in about 10% of the time allowed for inpatient care.[13]

The quality assessment plan must address the question: "What do nurses in the outpatient surgery area do for patients?" or "What is the scope of practice?" This can include preoperative preparation, postoperative comfort, recognition and prevention of postoperative complications, and patient/family education. All these activities must be addressed in a very short time.

Patients in the outpatient setting are at risk because of the brevity of time spent under the care of the professional health care staff. A major risk management concern is that adequate preoperative and postoperative teaching are performed to minimize adverse outcomes after surgery. Is the patient/family competent to provide necessary follow-up care in the home? Is a home care referral needed to maximize quality care for a positive outcome? Has the procedure been explained clearly to the patient before signing the operative consent? Is this a high-risk patient that might be more safely addressed in the acute setting? Are medication allergies properly identified?

Utilization management again is concerned with appropriate use of resources. Is the outpatient setting the appropriate level of care for this patient? If this procedure is unsafe for this particular patient, though the surgery itself can be performed safely in the outpatient setting, are necessary resources being underutilized? Many insurance companies only pay for certain surgeries if performed in the outpatient setting. However, an astute nurse practicing integrated quality management may determine this as inappropriate utilization for this particular patient. With adequate reasons, payors will waive the rules to provide patient safety.

The outpatient surgery patient is a candidate for infection because of the return to the home, a noncontrolled environment, or because of inadequate preoperative teaching. A common concern is postoperative pneumonia because the patient failed to understand the importance of inhalation therapy to expand the lungs after anesthesia, which is especially true if the patient is sent home on narcotics for pain control. Although patients are instructed to ambulate after discharge, pain and discomfort may hamper recovery unless the patient and family understand the consequent adverse outcomes. Inadequate patient/family teaching may result in a hospital admission that could have been prevented, a utilization management problem.

Again the outpatient nurse has less time to provide integrated quality management than the acute, long-term care, or home care nurse. The nurse may never see the patient again after discharge. In only a few hours the nurse must complete a nursing assessment that includes quality assessment, utilization management, infection control, and risk and safety management. Even in a "short-stay" environment, the outpatient nurse can make a positive impact on patient care through integrated quality management.

❖ IMPLICATIONS OF INTEGRATED QUALITY MANAGEMENT FOR PROFESSIONAL NURSING PRACTICE

Professional nurses have both the right and the responsibility to participate in integrated quality management. The nursing administrator benefits through increased organizational efficiency and cost reduction. There is the added advantage of regulatory compliance because the components of quality are mandated by both JCAHO and Medicare regulations. However, there are many other reasons to integrate quality management into nursing practice:

1. Increased visibility and effectiveness for nurses
2. Added recognition for nurses as competent, quality-conscious professionals

3. Gained power to be proactive in problem solving
4. More chart review and feedback leading to better documentation
5. Improved communication
6. Shared information
7. Less fragmentation in continuity of care
8. Less energy and resources spent in duplication

The end result of integrating quality management processes into all levels of nursing practice in all settings is improved patient care outcomes and empowerment of nurses as key professionals in health care quality.

REFERENCES

1. Barmann K, Domask M: A multidisciplinary approach: assuring quality of care for the diabetic client, *Journal of Nursing Quality Assurance* 3(2):19–25, 1989.
2. Bush D: *Quality management through statistics . . . the next quality assurance generation*, Blackwood, NJ, 1989-1990, Diversified Business Associates.
3. Etzwiler D: Inpatient and outpatient hospital-based diabetes education programs, *Practical Diabetology* 6:1–3, 1987.
4. Fitzpatrick JJ, Whall AL: *Conceptual models of nursing*, Bowie, Md, 1983, Prentice-Hall.
5. Hebelin K: Components of a quality assessment and assurance program, *Contemporary Long Term Care*, p 70, May 1988.
6. Ishikawa K: *Guide to quality control*, Asian Productivity Organization, p 24–26.
7. Home infusion therapy's bright prospects, *Jenks Healthcare Business Report* 1(4):1, 1990.
8. McCann J: Long-term home care for the elderly: perceptions of nurses, physicians, and primary caregivers, *Qual Rev Bull*, p 66, March 1988.
9. McManis G: Challenges of new decade demand break with tradition, *Modern Healthcare* 20(1): 60, 1990.
10. Neuman B: *The Neuman systems model: application to nursing education and practice*, New York, 1982, Appleton-Century-Crofts.
11. Neuman B: *The Betty Neuman model: a total person approach to patient problems*. In Riehl JP, Roy C, editors: *Conceptual models for nursing practice*, New York, 1980, Appleton-Century-Crofts.
12. *The New Webster's Medical Dictionary*, Lewtan Line, Hartford, Conn, 1988.
13. Synder L: QA in an outpatient surgery center, *Journal of Quality Assurance* 11(4): 9–11, 1989.
14. *Webster's New World Dictionary of American Language*, college edition, Cleveland and New York, 1986, World Publishing.

CHAPTER

10

❖

Implications for Collaborative Practice with Other Disciplines

❖ INTRODUCTION

Health care professionals face problems so complex that no one discipline can address them all. In fact few of the current health care issues can be solved without more than one discipline's professional expertise. Some of the societal issues faced today include the growing older adult population with chronic illnesses, the spread of AIDS, substance abuse, adolescent pregnancy, the growing population of uninsured and indigent, the homeless, and victims of violence. In such crises as these only a comprehensive approach to health care can be effective. This approach demands interdisciplinary collaboration.[11]

Throughout health care history, attempts have been made to produce an interdisciplinary approach to patient care. The JCAHO and Medicare regulations state that in certain areas, such as in the critical care, long-term care, psychiatric services, substance abuse services, and rehabilitation setting, interdisciplinary quality assessment and improvement is mandatory. Evidence of this is reviewed at each survey time. In fact if it could be regulated, interdisciplinary collaboration would be present today as these regulations cover many areas of varied disciplines' practice. To make this necessary concept a reality, education about what the concept is and what helps or hinders this process may be helpful.

❖ COLLABORATION: BY DEFINITION

Collaborative practice has become a frequently used word in recent health care journals. Some simply define *collaboration* as the art of working together. Webster defines *collaborate* as "to labor together . . . to work jointly with others especially in an intellectual endeavor . . . to cooperate with an agency with which one is not immediately connected . . ."[18] Baggs and Schmitt define *collaboration* by identifying key attributes needed, such as ". . . sharing in planning, making decisions, solving problems, setting goals and assuming responsibility; . . . coordinating . . . communicating openly. . . ."[2]

When applied directly to health care, *collaborative practice* means ". . . working together in a cooperative venture that recognizes the expertise of each health profession."[14] Weiss and Davis define *collaboration* as "interactions . . . that enable the knowledge and skills of . . . professionals to synergistically influence patient care being provided."[19] The American Nurses Association defined *collaboration* as follows[1]:

> Collaboration means true partnership, in which the power on both sides is valued by both, with recognition and acceptance of separate and combined spheres of activity and responsibility, mutual safeguarding of the legitimate interest of each party, and a commonality of goals that is recognized by both parties. This is a relationship based upon recognition that each is richer and more truly real because of the strength and uniqueness of the other.

Collaboration is a process that, given the opportunity, can produce a synergistic result: a positive outcome that no one discipline could have attained alone. Without a doubt, collaborative practice is something each discipline must embrace and sustain if quality patient care outcomes are to become reality in today's complex health care environment.

❖ INTERDISCIPLINARY: BY DEFINITION

Webster defines *interdisciplinary* as ". . . involving two or more academic, scientific, or artistic disciples."[18] *Discipline* is defined as ". . . a field of study . . . a rule or system of rules governing conduct or activity. . . .";[18] Other words such as *multidisciplinary, crossdisciplinary,* or *transdisciplinary* are often used interchangeably. Scott wrote, "Interdisciplinarity is plagued with misunderstandings about terminology . . ."[17] To understand the term, one must review who makes up this group.

Professionals strive for expert knowledge in their scientific area. Their continued development as experts produces specialized knowledge and skills. Although this has positive aspects, Kockelmans sees the specialization that has been the theme for more than 200 years as "the predominant trend in research and education . . ." leading to ". . . dangerous fragmentation . . . our theoretical knowledge has disintegrated . . . the human personality . . . affected by this lack of integration."[7]

Schein further explains the problem of integration versus specialization as resulting in certain professionals who are unable to look at issues holistically. Total system concepts that could be articulated among interconnected areas of traditional responsibility have been reduced to "conceptual boundaries that exist between disciplines."[16] No adequate theory of interdisciplinary groups in human service has been created.[11]

Before interdisciplinary collaboration can occur, expectations of the involved disciplines must be defined. This can empower the group as a unified team to move in the same direction, to commit to common objectives, and to focus on integrated outcomes. Otherwise confusion and fragmentation will result.

❖ FACTORS THAT PROMOTE OR HINDER INTERDISCIPLINARY COLLABORATIVE PRACTICE

Interdisciplinary collaboration in quality management does not occur simply by bringing a group of professionals together in one place. A highly diverse, interdisciplinary group gathered together will not necessarily make a cohesive team, regardless of their professional skills. Certain factors must be present. Devereux describes three components necessary in the delivery of quality patient care in interdisciplinary collaboration. These are "communication, competence, and accountability."[5]

Communication is important as each tries to understand the perspective of the other as assessed from each discipline's unique point of view. **Competence** is essential to build a level of trust among participating professionals so they feel they can rely on the other's knowledge and skills. **Accountability** is a cornerstone to effective collaborative practice because it implies "the ability to assume responsibility for one's own practice, taking ownership for one's decisions and actions . . . a level of professional maturity. . . ."[15]

Other factors that also need consideration are cooperativeness and assertiveness. Another is receptivity and respect for each other's professional contributions. Another essential skill is the ability to negotiate. Organizational factors such as administrative support can enhance or hinder collaborative practice.[15] According to Mariano three factors will either promote or hinder interdisciplinary collaborative practice[11]: (1) role and goal conflict; (2) decision making; and (3) communication.

In an interdisciplinary group several goals must be considered. First, there are patient, professional, and organizational goals. These can be either long or short term. Later, task and maintenance goals must be decided.[11]

Certain functions such as agreement on the priorities and actions to be taken can be agreed on, with specific outcomes defined if goals are stated clearly. This will reduce goal conflict that can arise from value differences, and it will promote team functioning. Value differences result from differing philosophies, beliefs, or professional socialization. These should be honestly discussed in a way that is nonthreatening if trust is to develop among team members. Quality management processes may call for some value judgments and may promote discussion. Focusing on defined goals such as safe and effective patient care can assist in developing consensus and maintaining group purpose.

Role conflict can hinder interdisciplinary collaboration in quality management. Sometimes there are overlapping responsibilities or abilities and competencies. Stereotyping can hinder group function, so it is important that each discipline understand the contribution to collaborative practice each discipline has to offer. Each discipline must teach the other about its skills and knowledge base. Team members can verbalize their strengths and weaknesses to the group so that each can better compliment the other. Ducanis and Golin state that a good exercise to reduce role conflict is to have interdisciplinary team members to (1) clarify role perceptions and expectations of each other; (2) identify each other's competencies as well as their own; (3) investigate overlapping roles and responsibilities; and (4) renegotiate role responsibilities as they relate to a specific group.[6]

Decision making can have a definite effect on interdisciplinary team effectiveness. To produce a positive team outcome, the problem must be clearly defined, the members' roles decided, and options and alternatives must be thoroughly discussed. This can decrease duplication and fragmentation in interdisciplinary collaborative practice.

Communication is necessary to promote effectiveness in interdisciplinary collaboration. Members must share their ideas and aspirations, including disagreements and feedback that is honest and constructive. Communication should convey an element of trust in an atmosphere that is "safe" and without retaliation for effective collaboration. This is crucial to team effectiveness.

❖ BENEFITS TO NURSING AND PATIENT CARE

When nursing reaches out to other disciplines for input and collaboration in integrated quality management, improved patient care outcomes result. For this to occur, the organizational climate and administrative support for interdisciplinary collaboration must be pervasive in the health care setting.

Disciplines that may be included in collaborative practice include, but are not limited to, physicians, pharmacists, respiratory, physical, and occupational therapists, dietitians, medical social workers, laboratory professionals, radiology professionals, and chaplains. Depending on the setting any or all of these disciplines may have a direct impact on the quality care a patient receives. Collaborative practice must focus on providing high quality patient care in a cost-efficient way.

Benefits of collaborative practice are documented in various literature. The National Joint Practice Commission study projects some benefits to be "(1) improved job stability and satisfaction for nurses, (2) improved quality of patient care, (3) increased patient satisfaction, and (4) reduced costs to the institution."[10] A study of collaborative practice at Hartford Hospital in Connecticut indicated one primary benefit: facilitating quality patient care. However, other benefits were increased autonomy and decision making, increased job satisfaction, and increased communications.[8]

Benefits such as these would predictably coincide in collaborative practice in integrated quality management. As interdisciplinary communication increases through collaborative practice, patient care problems can be identified earlier. Redundant questions resulting from overlapping roles in quality management can be eliminated, thereby minimizing wasted professional time and energy. Through the sharing of each discipline's unique viewpoint, synergistic approaches to solutions would create more positive patient care outcomes. Nursing would experience another point of view: one that must be valued as different but influential on the patient care outcome. The essence of collaborative practice is the "mutual exchange, integration, and use of ideas which lead to an optimal patient care process and outcome."[12]

Other positive outcomes have also been recorded in the nursing literature. Whitney identified several benefits of collaborative practice for nursing. These include the following[20]: (1) improvement in documenting the cost effectiveness and quality of nursing care, (2) development and implementation of new health care delivery systems through research and theory, (3) preparation for leadership in the future, and (4) development of new ways to measure quality and evaluate performance. These are some key benefits to remember as nursing initiates collaborative practice in quality management.

❖ STRATEGIES FOR COLLABORATIVE PRACTICE

Similarities, not differences, among disciplines must be highlighted. The quality management goal of providing positive patient outcomes must be kept in the forefront while the various disciplines collaborate on problems facing patient care delivery. Quality patient care outcomes are a concern for all health care professionals.

One way to enhance collaborative practice is to create an atmosphere that is creative and responsive by starting with small, achievable projects. When successful, the various disciplines will be more likely to tell others and offer to participate in the next quality management activity. Always keep a specific goal in mind while the interdisciplinary team addresses a quality management problem. No professional wants to waste energy committing to projects that do not have a specific, defined goal.

If the interdisciplinary team decides to meet, start promptly. A professional's time is valuable, and both being on time and starting on time builds trust and credibility among professionals. Perhaps various disciplines can rotate chairing these meetings to further enhance group ownership and collaboration.

Integrated care records may be used to develop collaborative practice among disciplines, providing a formal record of interdisciplinary communication, a factor that is needed to promote collaboration. This is especially important as regulatory agencies look at records for interdisciplinary quality assessment.

Development of an interdisciplinary quality management group, whose purpose would be to "identify problems, derive mutually satisfactory solutions, and learn more about the work and perspectives of one another,"[13] would promote joint practice. Problem process identification and resolution through quality improvement are the intents of quality management, and such a practice group would promote collaboration. A task that might be given such a group is to review the quality and appropriateness of patient care in a case study.

As mentioned earlier the medical record is the chief document for review of patient care. An interdisciplinary chart review would enhance collaborative practice and improve patient care outcomes because members could discuss the care together and share concerns. Record review is especially important to new professionals as they become familiar with the importance that documentation has in professional practice. Perhaps attending an interdisciplinary record review meeting could be part of each nurse's orientation.

For collaborative practice to occur, professionals may need help in developing the skills needed for collaboration. Special educational opportunities for all disciplines might include assertiveness training, change theory, communication skills, and professional attitude development. These are not always part of professional education. Furthermore, if various disciplines are to collaborate on quality management issues, they must attend classes and read the same literature necessary for nurses to understand the concept and put it into practice.

❖ EXAMPLES OF COLLABORATIVE PRACTICE IN QUALITY MANAGEMENT

Quality patient outcomes are an essential goal for all health care professionals. Delivery of health care services often involves more than one discipline. Therefore processes must be in place to afford collaboration for effective problem identification and solution among disciplines. As stated previously, interdisciplinary teams can consist of, but are not limited to, physicians, nurses, pharmacists, radiology and laboratory professionals, social services, dietitians, and physical, respiratory, speech, and/or occupational therapists. In some settings there are also nursing assistants or radiology assistants who also are a part of the quality management interdisciplinary team.

Examples of Collaborative Practice

An example of collaborative practice is one identified by the University of Wisconsin Hospital and Clinics (UWHC) in Madison, Wisconsin. Laboratory professionals and critical care nurses formed a focus team to establish quality requirements for specimen collection and labeling. Of the 50,000 specimens received each month, approximately one half were collected by laboratory personnel and the other half by nursing and medical personnel. Plagued by a consistent number of incorrect or incomplete specimen labels, the laboratory identified mislabeling as a quality problem affecting patient care.

A utilization management problem occurred when incorrectly labeled specimens had to be recollected, with rework and inefficient use of both collectors and laboratory processors. More important, the patient treatment was delayed because of late laboratory results. There was risk because a patient could receive the wrong treatment if incorrect data were charted because of mislabeling. Each recollection required an additional needle stick, putting the patient at risk for infection. The laboratory set up a quality assurance (assessment) study to have proper specimen labeling 100% of the time.

The three types of mislabeling that most often occurred were: (1) the specimen form was not labeled or did not have complete patient information; (2) the patient information on the specimen did not correspond to the request form; and (3) the label appeared correct, but the ordering source reported the name on the label did not correspond with the patient from whom the specimen was collected. With careful monitoring of the system for 3 months, staff determined that the majority of mislabeling occurred when nonlaboratory personnel collected the specimen.

Next the quality specimen requirements were submitted to the nursing QA committee for endorsement of joint responsibility in this problem. Because it is the accepted practice at UWHC that blood from ICU patients be collected only by nursing or medical personnel, and 45% of the mislabeling came from the ICU area, this area became part of the unit-based QA committee's monitoring and evaluation processes. Together, the laboratory and nursing and medicine were able to identify three steps toward corrective action: (1) identify all quality requirements for all medical and nursing personnel, (2) assign prestamped patient labels for ICU patients with a mechanism to double-check for accuracy with ICU support staff, and (3) provide a central location at which the specimen collection container could be found.

Although initially each discipline collected its own QA data, management from each area recommended forming a focus group with each discipline represented. This allowed the laboratory and ICU nurses to discuss any needed improvement of quality processes in an open and direct manner on a regular basis. Results included the following[9]: (1) increased awareness of mislabeling and the effect this had on patient care delivery; (2) refinement of the mutual monitoring process; (3) more effective, open communication; and (4) more respect for the roles of each discipline in providing patient care.

As a result of this collaborative practice in QM, an ICU nursing/laboratory form was developed for problem identification. A transfer service was established to speed the delivery of specimens and get faster returns. Mutual tours of the working environments were conducted as each discipline learned more about the other. Shared education programs developed both skills and knowledge necessary for collaborative practice. No longer was communication one way; barriers between nursing and the laboratory were removed. Quality management plans were integrated rather than managed independently in one area. This model of integrated interdisciplinary quality management encouraged collaborative behaviors that resulted in personnel satisfaction, as well as improved patient care service.[9]

Interdisciplinary quality management can result in a positive patient outcome in discharge planning. In any setting several disciplines are responsible for determining the appropriate level of care for the patient and the appropriate setting for that care. Utilization management is part of discharge planning because each patient's needs are reviewed by several disciplines. The physician evaluates the patient's condition and when the patient can safely move to another level of care, for example, from hospital to home. The nurses assess the patient's needs for discharge teaching and home care nursing needs. The medical social worker assesses and determines the safety of the home environment and the support systems available to help with patient recovery. They also review the financial resources available to the patient.

The dietitian assesses the patient's nutritional status, a necessary component for healing, and provides that education as indicated. If the patient was seen by other therapists, such as speech or respiratory, those professionals would evaluate continued needs and refer those for home care follow-up. Often a patient is discharged on new and complicated medications with the risk of side effects; the pharmacist becomes a member of the discharge planning team. Home medical equipment must be ordered and delivered before patient arrival at home. Home care nurses must be informed and prepared to manage any infectious patient who is discharged to the home. Indeed the discharge planning team is truly an example of interdisciplinary collaborative practice.

Safety and risk factors are part of the discharge planning process. The medical equipment must be set up and functioning properly, or an adverse patient outcome could occur. Dietary education is crucial to management of many chronic illnesses such as diabetes; inefficient education or delay in education can cause the patient to experience an adverse outcome and possible readmission to the hospital. Medications must be clearly labeled and education provided to minimize the risks associated with pharmacologic agents. Continued inpatient treatment when not appropriate can increase the patient's risk of infection and falls that can occur in the hospital. Clearly the discharge planning process is one that lends itself well to interdisciplinary collaboration in quality management. As collaborative teams identify processes that can enhance discharge planning, improvement in the quality of the process with resulting improved patient outcomes can occur.

Another example of interdisciplinary collaborative practice in quality management is centered around a standard of surgical practice. It is standard to give preoperative antibiotics to certain patients, and it is accepted practice that the infusion must be complete before incision time. This is accomplished through the interrelated workings of several professionals. The surgeon orders the preoperative medication. The pharmacist provides the correct drug in the correct dosage and dilution. The nurse administers the medication before sending the patient to surgery. The anesthesiologist and circulating nurse must be sure the drug has infused before incision for the drug to be effective. This process must be collaborative to minimize the breaks that can occur.

Community Memorial Hospital in Menomonee Falls, Wisconsin, began a quality review of surgical patients who developed postoperative infections. This case review demonstrated that often there was incomplete infusion of the prophylactic medication before the incision. The surgeons thought it was caused by the nurses' delay in starting the medication process. The nurses explained that the delay was caused by either a delay in delivery from the pharmacy or a dilution volume that was too large to infuse before the incision time. Another complicating factor was that the patients were usually same day surgery patients who were admitted 2 hours before surgery, and the infusion had to occur 30 to 60 minutes before incision to be effective.

The nursing quality assurance (assessment) committee monitored any breakdowns for specifics. Data collected included whether the surgeon's order was verbal or standing, where the infusion actually began, the type of antibiotic ordered, time begun and completed, and time of incision. After a 2 week review the results showed that the standard was not met, with only 15% of the cases completing infusion 30 to 60 minutes before incision time.

After continued study staff discovered that each discipline was responsible for certain factors in failing to meet the standard. Some surgeons gave verbal orders in the operating room, and when surgery was ahead of schedule, the antibiotic did not have time to infuse. The pharmacy would deliver the drugs to several sites depending on when the drug was ordered and where it was begun. This was confusing and delayed infusion. The infection control committee assisted as the nurses learned that some antibiotics needed too large a volume for proper dilution and patients complained of burning if the medication infused too rapidly. Thus the patient's time for infusion extended past the time indicated for incision to begin. The collaborative approach allowed all disciplines to see where each could improve its practice for a better patient outcome. Changes were made in each area of practice as each took responsibility for its part in quality management.[4] The processes of care for these patients were improved as collaborative teamwork became reality.

❖ IMPLEMENTING QUALITY IMPROVEMENT TEAMS: AN OPPORTUNITY FOR INTERDISCIPLINARY COLLABORATION

The National Demonstration Project (NDP) has many examples of collaborative practice through continuous quality improvement. In one example Kaiser-Permanente addressed the problem of nonavailability of patient charts from the emergency room visit to the follow-up appointment area in ambulatory care. The team did not seek more staff, more money, or more equipment, which was often the answer to any problem. Instead, they designed a new process. The goals of the improved process were to (1) identify the patient's ambulatory care facility and (2) get the emergency room record delivered there.

A flow diagram was used to define the importance of each part of the process to make it successful (Fig. 10-1). The team found that unnecessary information was delivered by some departments and inadequate information delivered by others. The flow diagram helped all team members to see how they were customers in some cases and suppliers in others (Fig. 10-2). For example, the emergency department was the supplier of valuable information needed for subsequent treatment of the patient.

Then a cause-and-effect diagram was developed by the team. After brainstorming the basic causes for the inefficient process were related to six areas: labeling, copying, arrival, identifying information, sorting, and trans-

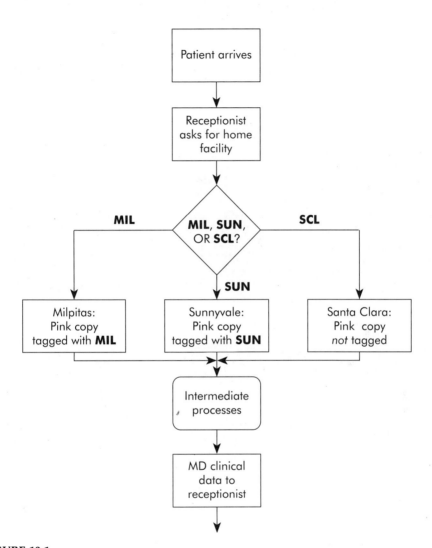

FIGURE 10-1
A, Initial description of record transfer process: a process flow diagram (Kaiser-Permanente Project).

150 INTEGRATED QUALITY MANAGEMENT

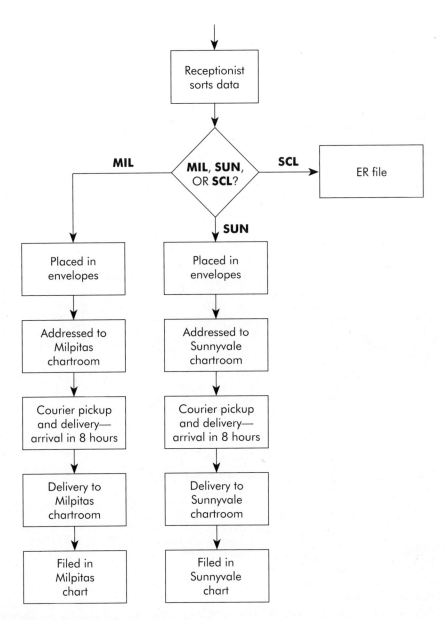

FIGURE 10-1 (continued).
B, Initial description of record transfer process: a process flow diagram (Kaiser-Permanente Project). (From Berwick DM et al: *Curing health care: new strategies for quality improvement*, San Francisco, 1990, Jossey-Bass, pp. 226–227.)

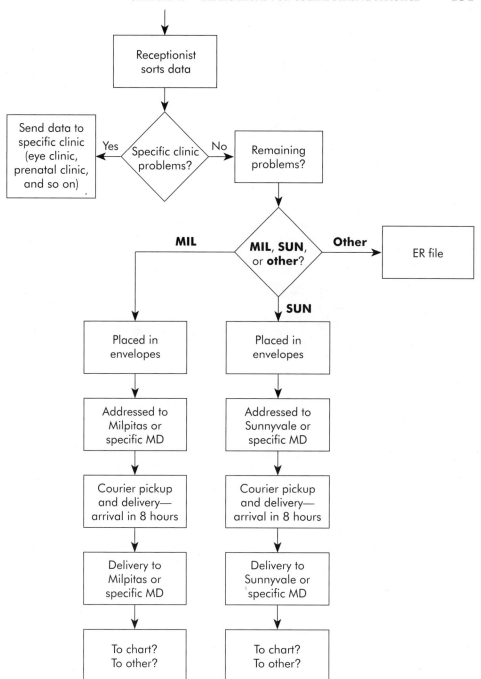

FIGURE 10-2
A, Revised description of record transfer process: a process flow diagram (Kaiser-Permanente Project).

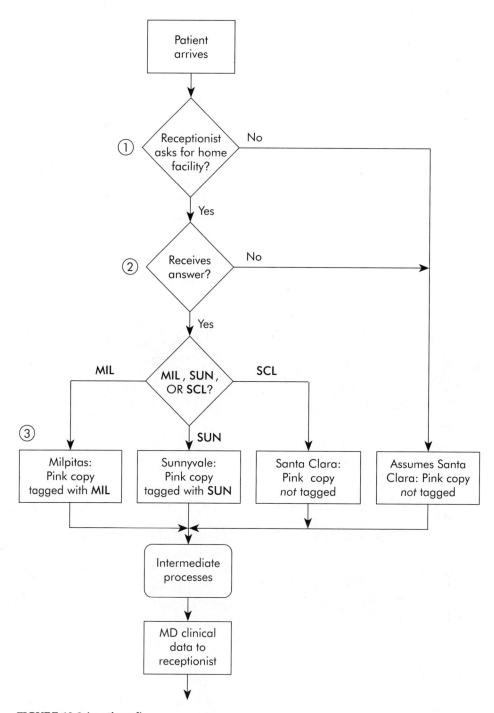

FIGURE 10-2 (continued).
B, Revised description of record transfer process: a process flow diagram (Kaiser-Permanente Project). (From Berwick DM et al: *Curing health care: new strategies for quality improvement*, San Francisco, 1990, Jossey-Bass, pp. 228–229.)

fer. Each has several possible explanations for the specific error (Fig. 10-3).

Berwick states that, once the quality improvement team has determined the diagnosis of the problem, three steps must take place[3]: (1) develop the remedy, (2) implement and test the remedy, and (3) deal with the resistance to change.

Different members of the quality improvement team have unique understandings of the process under study. The strength of this team is that different solutions may be suggested. When the approach is evaluated for determining priority, cost and time needed (utilization management) and the mechanism to monitor and evaluate effectiveness (quality assessment and improvement) must be defined. The team, rather than a singular department, can make these decisions more effectively.

Berwick gives several guidelines for successful implementation of the remedies[3]:

1. Encourage participation.
   Those most likely to be affected by the change should be on the team. This can minimize conflict at a later time.
2. Provide enough time.
   Project solutions risk more from moving too quickly than from progressing slowly. This allows for team members to get to know each other and allows time to build trust.
3. Keep the project focused.
   Projects with a narrow scope are the most successful. This encourages the team to focus on getting results.
4. Work closely with leadership.
   Leadership should be active in all quality improvement team processes, but this is especially important in the implementation phase.
5. Treat everyone with dignity.
   Change is not easy for anyone. In interdisciplinary teamwork, change can be viewed as indicative of a "problem" or that someone was doing something wrong. Remember, quality improvement teams are developed to fix a process, not to blame anyone.

At Kaiser-Permanente the quality improvement team members, through collaborative, interdisciplinary practice, developed a better understanding of the existing processes for transfer of the emergency room record to the various ambulatory clinics for patient follow-up. The team identified flaws in the present process and designed a new, effective process using existing resources. The solution included using the available computer systems more efficiently and tagging the chart for the appropriate follow-up clinic site. The

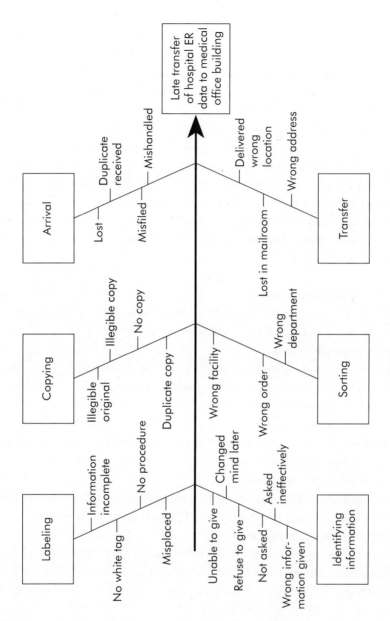

FIGURE 10-3
Cause-and-effect diagram for timely transfer of emergency room records to satellite medical office building (Kaiser-Permanente Project). (From Berwick DM et al: *Curing health care: new strategies for quality improvement*, San Francisco, 1990, Jossey-Bass, p. 231.)

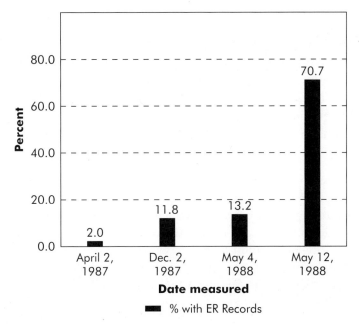

FIGURE 10-4
Santa Clara emergency room records found in Milpitas charts (Kaiser-Permanente Project). (From Berwick DM et al: *Curing health care: new strategies for quality improvement*, San Francisco, 1990, Jossey-Bass, p. 234.)

team implemented the new process effectively (Fig. 10-4). This is an example of effective integrated quality management. Resources were wasted through an inefficient process (utilization management). The patient, the external customer, might arrive for a follow-up visit, and the physician, the internal customer, would be unable to treat the patient appropriately without necessary record information (safety management). Documentation might not be as thorough and accurate without the prior record as a guide (risk management). If the emergency department treated a patient for an infection, lack of record information at the clinic site could jeopardize effective follow-up treatment. This process is an excellent one for quality assessment and improvement.

❖ SUMMARY

Interdisciplinary quality management offers many opportunities to improve patient care outcomes as collaborative practice takes place in every health care setting. Nurses have much to offer as major players in collaborative patient care and integrated quality management. As health care continues to become more complex, interdisciplinary collaboration will be even more important to implement safe and effective health care solutions. As one nurse states[4]:

> Reality is that delivering quality patient care involves multiple disciplines and that our own practices are intertwined with responsibilities in achieving that standard of care. If a multidisciplinary quality assurance (assessment and improvement) approach is not used, those aspects of care will not be evaluated. Although multidisciplinary monitoring can be frustrating and time consuming because of the politics and interpersonal issues, it can also be the most rewarding in affecting actual patient care.

REFERENCES

1. American Nurses Association: Nursing: a social policy statement, Kansas City, 1980, ANA, p 7.
2. Baggs J, Schmitt M: Collaboration between nurses and physicians, *Image: The Journal of Nursing Scholarship* 20(3):145, 1988.
3. Berwick DM, Godfrey AB, Roessner J: *Curing health care: new strategies for quality improvement*, San Francisco, 1990, Jossey-Bass.
4. Brukakken K: Preoperative antibiotic adminsitration: a case for interdisciplinary monitoring, *J Nurs Qual Assur* 3(2):69–73, 1989.
5. Devereux P: Does joint practice work? *J Nurs Adm* 11(6):40, 1981.
6. Ducanis AJ, Golin AK: *The interdisciplinary and health care team handbook*, Germantown, Md, 1979, Aspen Publishers.
7. Kockelmans JJ: *Why interdisciplinarity? interdisciplinarity and higher education*, University Park, Pa, 1979, Pennsylvania State University Press.
8. Koerner B, Cohen J, Armstrong D: Professional behavior in collaborative practice, *J Nurs Adm* 16(10):39–43, 1986.
9. Kohles M, Barry P: Clinical laboratory and nursing personnel: collaboration in improving patient care, *J Nurs Qual Assur* 3(2):1–10, 1989.
10. Kuhn R: Nurse and physician collaboration: how to strenghten the team, *Heart Lung* 14(4):82, 1985.
11. Mariano C: The case for interdisciplinary collaboration, *Nursing Outlook* 37(6):285, 1989.
12. Mills M: The CNS and collaborative practice, *Clinical Nurse Specialist* 4(4):194, 1990.

13. Notkin MS: Collaboration and communication, *Nursing Administration Quarterly*, p 4, Fall 1983.
14. Oulton JA: Collaboration—at what price? *The Canadian Nurse* 85(7), 1989 (editorial).
15. Puta D: Nurse-physician collaboration toward quality, *J Nurs Qual Assur* 3(2):15, 1989.
16. Schein E: *Professional education, the Carnegie commission on higher education*, New York, 1972, McGraw-Hill.
17. Scott R: *Personal and institutional problems encountered in being interdisciplinary*. In Kockelmans JJ, editor: *Interdisciplinary and Higher Education*, University Park, Pa, 1979, Pennsylvania State University Press.
18. *Webster's New Collegiate Dictionary*, Springfield, Mass, 1981, G & C Merriam.
19. Weiss SL, Davis HP: Validity and reliability of collaborative practice scales, *Nurs Res* 34(5):299, 1985.
20. Whitney FW: An economic view of collaboration between nursing service and education, *Nurs Econ* 4:37–42, 1986.

CHAPTER

11

Quality Management in Acute Care

❖ HISTORY OF ACUTE CARE HOSPITALS

THE development and growth of acute care hospitals in the United States can be divided into five distinct periods. The word *hospital* comes from the Latin root word *hostel*, which in the Middle Ages meant refuge for the sick, poor, and weary. The first hospitals were mostly charitable and religious in origin. In the United States the first hospitals were infirmaries in poorhouses. An example is Charity Hospital in New Orleans, which was established in 1736 and is still operating today. Private voluntary hospitals, supported by community leaders, date back to the eighteenth century. Massachusetts General Hospital in Boston was established as a private voluntary hospital in 1873. By 1873 approximately 178 private voluntary hospitals were operating throughout the United States.[3]

The first growth period for hospitals occurred between 1870 and 1910. This period is noted for the development of biomedical and technical interventions to improve health, such as surgery with anesthesia. By 1909 the number of hospitals had increased to 4300. Many of these hospitals were for-profit organizations owned and operated by physicians. Medical care became more complicated and required more specialized knowledge and equipment.

Between 1910 and 1945 hospitals reflected new medical discoveries such as the treatment of infectious diseases with antibiotics. Pernicious anemia was treated with liver extract. Insulin was discovered, and diabetes treatment was revolutionized. Rehabilitation hospitals became popular, bringing disabled persons to the hospital setting. More chronic illness patients came to the hospitals for treatment. This period guaranteed hospitals a place in health care delivery.

By 1945 growth, influenced by several factors, began again. The insurance business took on a new look with Blue Cross/Blue Shield, which was developed during the Depression and was designed to protect the hospital and physician from loss of payment. Medical services expanded both in intensity and type. The Hill-Burton Act encouraged rural hospital expansion by providing federal funds to allow access to health care in rural areas. Hospitals developed diploma nursing programs to meet the increased demands for professional staff. In 1965 the federal government started the Medicare program to provide health care to the elderly population of the United States. The Medicaid program also was defined, extending health care to the poor. All of these factors empowered the acute care setting, the hospital, with growth opportunities.

Today hospitals are still big business and demand the largest portion of health care reimbursement. Many multi-hospital systems have developed as health care dollars are more competitive; some small hospitals have closed as a result. This is still the primary health care delivery system in the United States and provides many jobs for Americans, especially nurses.

❖ ACUTE CARE IN THE 1990s

Many economic and demographic changes are influencing the acute care setting in the 1990s. The older population is becoming larger with the fastest growing segment of the population being more than 85 years of age. This group is primarily dependent on Medicare for health care coverage in acute care and consumes the majority of health care resources available. The hospital administration is seeing this part of its patient mix grow, with restricted reimbursement from the government. Managed care is more prevalent with attention given to cost-effective, quality care for the privately insured.

The acute care facility of the 1990s will depend on proactive, innovative management. Even in a shrinking market the acute care organization can move the facility into the 1990s with confidence. Key components of proactive management that acute care managers must incorporate are strategic planning, strengthening referral bases, collaborating with other acute care hospitals, meeting community needs, and continuously improving quality. The acute care hospital that is known for its quality is less susceptible to the fluctuations in economy and reimbursement as its customers express their preference by use of services. To implement the strategic plan and provide quality patient care, acute care managers must identify key strategic initiatives, including defining internal and external customers and developing a process for quality improvement. This means constantly assessing the organization's performance and evaluating where improvements can occur. Continuous quality improvement is necessary for the acute care setting to continue to survive in the 1990s.[4]

❖ QUALITY MANAGEMENT IN ACUTE CARE: UNIQUE ISSUES

Just like every other health care setting, acute care facilities are being critically analyzed by consumers, insurance companies, and accrediting agencies to demonstrate the "quality" of their services. Requests for information and data by external agencies are a norm. The hospital is charged with developing information management systems and analyzing data for validity, reliability, as well as usefulness to the organization. The acute care facility must also prioritize the data collection to analyze needs, because this is labor intensive and thus costly.

To demonstrate the value of acute care services, the hospital must act responsibly in defining quality indicators and compare data for opportunities for quality improvement. Quality indicators most common to acute care are nosocomial infection, mortality, and readmission rates. Infection rates in the hospital might include surgical wounds, sepsis, urinary tract infections, and respiratory tract infections. Unplanned returns to surgery and quality assessment and improvement study results are important in evaluating quality in the acute care setting. Other utilization indicators include average length of stay and cost per service or procedure for the patients with specific diseases.

Quality assessment extends to the professionals providing the health care services. Accrediting agencies want to know the competency of the medical staff and how each is credentialed. Is there evidence of continuing education and training? Nurses are also reviewed as to ratios of RN to LPN to nursing assistants. Personnel files of management and staff are reviewed for credentials and evidence of both competency and continuing education. Nurse-to-patient ratios are important data as are the numbers of nurses with BSNs and MSNs. What ongoing monitoring and evaluating processes are in place for quality assessment and improvement in professional practice in hospitals?

More emphasis is placed on patient satisfaction survey results in the acute care setting. No longer is the satisfaction of the patient assumed. Now it is valued as an indicator of quality service. Also employer and employee satisfaction surveys are gaining popularity as the acute care management team involves staff in improving quality care. What the staff members think and how well they perform will affect the satisfaction of patients and consequently the quality of care provided.

❖ INTEGRATED CLINICAL QUALITY MANAGEMENT IN ACUTE CARE

As part of continuous quality improvement in acute care, nursing must look at integrating clinical quality management into the practice setting. The individual functions of clinical quality management have been in place in the acute care setting for some time. Often distinct practitioners are assigned to coordinate infection control, quality assessment, utilization management, and risk/safety management, both in the nursing division and house wide.

However, in integrated clinical quality management these philosophies and skills must be taken to the staff and nursing management levels. Because nurses are the primary care givers in the acute care setting 24 hours a day and provide most of the documentation of patient care and response, they must integrate quality management into daily nursing practice.

Peer Review Organization

The arm of the Health Care Financing Administration (HCFA) that reviews acute care records for quality concerns is the Peer Review Organization (PRO). Both professional staff and management must be familiar with the generic quality screens by which acute care records are reviewed. There are currently seven screens, the first being *adequacy of discharge planning*. Here the nurse reviewer is looking for documentation of appropriate planning for care of the patient who has left the hospital with respect to the patient's physical, mental, and emotional needs. Documentation required includes a needs assessment, development of a plan, and initiation of appropriate arrangements to provide a smooth transition to posthospital care. The plan should identify additional resources needed and provide adequate patient and family teaching. A failed screen is one in which there is no documentation. A confirmed quality problem is when the patient's needs were not met.[1]

The second screen is *medical stability of the patient*. The entire category describes "aberrant clinical data" that was either not recognized or inadequately treated while the patient was in the hospital. Here the nurse or physician reviewer looks for stable blood pressures, temperature no greater than 101°F, and no purulent or bloody drainage within 24 hours of discharge. Pulse must not be less than 50 or greater than 120 at 4 hours before discharge. Intravenous fluids or drugs must be complete by midnight the day of discharge. Also the reviewer looks for any abnormal diagnostic result or finding that has not been resolved by discharge. If any of these are present, the physician may use his or her judgment in discharging the patient and document why it is safe to do so. Evidence of actions taken must be documented in the record.

Screen three is *deaths*. This is especially noteworthy to the PRO reviewer if death occurred during or following a surgical procedure. A confirmed quality problem would be any recorded intraoperative or postoperative death resulting from inadequate preoperative assessment or improper procedures resulting from surgical or anesthesia complications. Any death occurring within 24 hours following return to a special care unit such as coronary care is reviewed. Any death that is unexpected is a red flag to reviewers of quality patient care. An unexplained death is defined as death occurring when reasonable expectation on admission was that the patient would recover.[1]

Next is screen four, *nosocomial infections*, or hospital acquired infections. A failed screen is not always a confirmed quality problem. The reviewer would declare a failed screen when one or more of the following is identified as an indicator of infection within 72 hours of admission to the acute care setting:

1. Oral temperature is 101°F or greater
2. Elevated WBC and/or left shift
3. Organism is isolated from body fluids or specimens
4. Productive cough
5. Dysuria, pyuria
6. Purulent drainage
7. Redness, heat, localized pain or tenderness
8. Radiologic imaging abnormalities

If two or more of these are present, the PRO reviewer will refer to the CDC guidelines to determine if indeed a nosocomial infection is defined. The presence of a nosocomial infection is a confirmed quality problem.[1]

Screen five is *unscheduled returns to surgery,* reviewing returns within the same admission for the same condition or to correct a surgical problem that occurred during the primary surgery. This is not limited to surgical procedures performed in the operating room. A surgical repair of a separated wound that is performed in the patient's room is considered an unscheduled return to surgery.

Screen six, *trauma suffered in the hospital,* is diverse. Here the reviewer looks for evidence of patient falls, serious complications of anesthesia, blood transfusion error or reaction, hospital acquired or deterioration of decubitus, or any serious complication resulting from lack of appropriate care. Unplanned return to surgery is again delineated with respect to surgery not specifically addressed in the surgical permit. Any medication error or adverse drug reaction with potential or actual harm is part of this screen.

Screen seven is called an *optional* screen. It addresses any change in treatment or medication, including discontinuing the drug, within 24 hours of discharge, without adequate observation. At any time a review of documentation, any unnecessary procedure, or any other concern can occur.

These generic quality screens address specific clinical quality management concerns including risk/safety, utilization, and infection control. A nurse administrator would use these screens to design some quality assessment indicators as well. Clearly the acute care nurse can benefit from understanding these PRO screens and the documentation required to address them in nursing practice.

Clinical Quality Management: Case Examples

Integrated clinical QM can be applied to any acute care patient from medical-surgical units to special care units to operating room care to obstetrics. The following are several case examples based on common acute care nursing patient needs.

Management of the Patient with Congestive Heart Failure. In any acute care setting the congestive heart failure (CHF) patient is a common visitor and repeater. This patient provides an excellent example of the positive impact that nursing can have when integrating clinical QM into the nursing practice. Several *quality assessment* indicators are appropriate for the CHF patient. When dealing with the CHF patient, it is important to monitor and evaluate shortness of breath, fluid retention, vital signs, and medication levels and response, such as digoxin, diuretics, anticoagulants, and potassium. Dietary monitoring is important for evaluating fluid and sodium intake.

Risk and safety management is crucial for the CHF patient. With multiple drugs ingested, a patient can experience side effects. A change in electrolyte balance can result in altered sensorium, as well as arrthymias when taking diuretics. This predisposes the patient to falls, as well as more serious side effects such as syncope or even death. Anticoagulants can have major adverse complications, and patients must be watched for drug interaction effects, as well as bleeding tendencies. For a CHF patient it is crucial to perform intake and output monitoring. Consistent weight monitoring is mandatory. Omission of this could result in an adverse outcome for the patient.

Infection control plays a major role in the care of the CHF patient. CHF patients are at high risk for skin breakdown because of dependent edema such as pedal edema. Skin ulcers can result. The CHF patient is also predisposed to pulmonary edema with consequent respiratory infections. The acute care nurse must be constantly aware how integrated infection control can affect quality management of the CHF patient.

There are many *utilization management* implications for the CHF patient in acute care. If any of the above complications occur, the CHF patient may have an increased length of stay in the hospital. Also these patients tend to have frequent admissions and readmissions. Comprehensive discharge planning and teaching are necessary for the CHF patient. Readmission can result from the patient's inability to manage medications at home. If the patient suffers from sensorium alteration, he or she may not take medications regularly or perhaps could experience a fall. If the taste of potassium is disagreeable, he or she may stop taking this drug, resulting in electrolyte and arrythmia problems.

Once back in a home environment the CHF patient may return to previous dietary habits that put him or her at high risk for readmissions. Truly the CHF patient has the potential to use excessive health care resources. Acute care patient education and home care follow-up are essential to clinical quality management in the CHF patient. QM improves self-care, maximizes outpatient services, and minimizes acute care readmissions.

Management of the Diabetic Patient. When dealing with a diabetic patient integrated clinical quality management is a must. This patient can have alterations in blood sugar, with both immediate and future adverse outcomes. *Quality assessment* of the diabetic patient could include monitoring and evaluating blood sugar levels, vital signs, skin integrity, and patient education. Dietary monitoring and evaluation is also appropriate because diet directly affects blood sugar.

The diabetic patient is a high *risk,* problem-prone patient, and *safety* is extremely important. If the patient does not get feedings and snacks on schedule, metabolic problems such as hypoglycemia become a risk, causing altered sensorium and resulting in falls, as well as other environmental hazards. One adverse outcome of unmanaged diabetes is peripheral neuropathy. When the patient is unable to sense heat and cold because of decreased circulation, heating pads and cold packs become dangerous. Another characteristic of unmanaged diabetes is retinal neuropathy. Patients with decreased visual acuity or blurred vision are more likely to fall, stumble, or hurt themselves. Shoes are a major concern because improperly fitting shoes can cause ulcers. Without proper foot care diabetic patients are at risk for infections that could lead to amputations.

Infection control is a major quality concern for diabetic patients. Diabetics are slow to heal because of the metabolic problems associated with the disease. It is more crucial than normal that diabetics be protected from breaks in skin integrity. At the same time many diabetics must inject insulin into their skin several times a day. Any break in skin integrity is an opportunity for infection. Rotating injection sites can minimize these problems.

Infections can also occur with skin ulcers because of peripheral neuropathy. With decreased circulation to the skin and hampered healing, a diabetic could die from skin ulcers. The same is true of insect bites such as mosquito bites. The diabetic is handicapped in healing more than the person without diabetes. Precautions must be taken to avoid breaks in skin integrity.

The diabetic patient has other *infection risks.* As the diabetic patient experiences glycosuria, urinary tract infections may be more common. Dehydration can occur with polyuria. Again healing is impeded. Chronic infections can directly affect the health of the diabetic, producing an adverse patient care outcome.

The diabetic patient can also present *utilization management* challenges. These multifaceted problems of diabetes can result in repeated hospitalizations for stabilization. If the diabetic develops infection while in the hospital, a longer length of stay can be encountered. If other safety problems such as falls or burns occur in the hospital, time spent there is extended. Any extended length of stay that could have been avoided through integrated quality management is a waste of valuable health care resources.

Part of *utilization management* is discharge planning and teaching. Patient education must address dietary management, as well as drug understanding, administration, and side effects of medications. Implications for long-term complications such as retinopathy, cardiomyopathy, peripheral neuropathy, arteriosclerosis, and kidney disease must be understood by patient and caregiver. Patients need to know that stress factors such as trauma, infection, cold, or tension can increase the need for insulin, and a doctor may need to be consulted. Signs and symptoms of hyperglycemia and hypoglycemia are crucial parts of patient and family education. Good skin and foot care are also important, as well as monitoring of blood sugar. Patient education can help patients manage their care at home and prevent readmission to the hospital. Home care follow-up is appropriate to ensure that the patient education taught in the acute care setting is practiced and reinforced at home.

Through QM diabetic patients can better manage the personal care needed for a healthful lifestyle. Infections can be minimized, and acute care admissions decreased. Patients can function more safely in the home environment. Continued monitoring and assessment of patients' diabetes control can occur through QM in the physician office and/or outpatient clinic. This will best use health care resources and minimize adverse patient care outcomes.

Continuous Quality Improvement: Eliminating Drug Errors in Acute Care Services

York Hospital demonstrated CQI in managing drug errors. A quality improvement team consisting of members of the pharmacy and therapeutics committee, medical executive committee, critical care committee, infection control, and intensive care nursing met to address drug errors. The drug studied was potassium chloride, given intravenously to millions of Americans each year for electrolyte imbalance and cardiovascular function. If the drug is improperly mixed or diluted, death can result. Even a small variation can cause a delay in patient recovery and increase length of stay in the acute care setting (utilization management). The team was formed when a lawsuit resulted in connection with administration of this drug (risk management).

The team first addressed the fact that the labels on the different vendor bottles looked similar to other drugs. Care must be taken to use the right drug. Second, if the bottles were left in the wrong place, they had more chance for wrong selection for use. Third, the drug must be mixed thoroughly, or it will pool in one area, and the wrong concentrate will result.

The team at York began by limiting the locations for the drug concentrate and limiting the persons authorized to use them. All potassium chloride bottles were removed from nursing units, recovery room, operating room, and critical care. Only premixed solutions were allowed in patient care areas. Physicians cannot order additions to bags in use; a new bag must be prepared with accurate concentrations. Stat requests are filled in 15 minutes whenever possible.

The program has been in place since June 1991, with no reported drug errors and no adverse outcomes. The program incurred no additional costs to any department and is an example in which a team was employed to improve patient care and minimize adverse outcomes through QM/QI.[2]

❖ SUMMARY

Several case examples of patients who can benefit from quality management and improvement in nursing practice in the acute care setting have been cited. As more patient care shifts to alternative care settings such as outpatient and home or long-term care, the acute care nurse may see the sickest patients who are unable to use alternative delivery settings. A professional nurse with expert quality management education and implementation ability for acute care practice is needed.

For this reason integrating clinical quality management components into the practice of each manager and staff nurse is necessary to face the challenge of the acute care setting of the 1990s.

The acute care nurse has the opportunity to provide quality assessment and improvement for hospitalized patients while minimizing infections and risks and using health care resources appropriately. The acute care nurse can actually influence a positive patient outcome and minimize an adverse patient care outcome through clinical quality management. In a time when hospitals question which resources to use and which services to keep, nursing can demonstrate worth through integrated clinical quality management in professional nursing practice.

REFERENCES

1. *Generic quality screens, Third scope of work,* August 1990, Mid-South Foundation for Medical Care.
2. Hospital's team effort eliminating drug errors, *Modern Healthcare,* Oct 7, 1991.
3. Jonas S: *Health care delivery in the United States,* New York, 1986, Springer.
4. Proactive executives: prospering in tough times. *Hospitals,* p. 22, March 20, 1991.

CHAPTER

12

Quality Management in Ambulatory Care

❖ INTRODUCTION

THE major health care setting for the 1990s is ambulatory care. In 1983 less than 12% of total acute care revenues came from the outpatient setting. In 1987 this increased to 23%.[1] In 1990 the acute care facilities that had diversified in ambulatory care increased revenues 40% to 60%. Predictions are that the revenue mix for diversified health care systems by 1995 will be 50% ambulatory care and 50% acute care.[8]

Because senior management must plan strategically for the future with long-term goals, as well as short-term goals, ambulatory care will continue to be at the forefront for the next 20 years. This will be necessary to compete in the marketplace in the 1990s. Any new opportunities for growth must be discovered and managed well for industry security. There are several ways of approaching the ambulatory care market.

❖ AMBULATORY DELIVERY SETTINGS
Hospital-Based Ambulatory Care

Hospital-based ambulatory care has been the traditional way to provide outpatient services. At present 67.5% of hospitals in the United States have outpatient departments. Emergency care is another ambulatory care service offered by 83.9% of hospitals. Ambulatory surgery services are offered by 83.8 percent of hospitals.[11] Other services that a hospital may offer include health promotions, home care, sports medicine, women's health, and diagnostic services. The advent of hospital delivered ambulatory care is truly affecting the U.S. health care system.

Freestanding Ambulatory Care

Ambulatory care services have attracted the health care industry's entrepreneurs. Today almost all services offered by outpatient departments at the hospital are also offered by freestanding facilities. Freestanding urgent care and primary care centers have increased from 300 in 1980 to more than 3000 in 1987. These freestanding delivery systems provided about 5 million visits in 1980 compared with 43 million visits in 1987. Despite their growth only 30% have remained financially viable.[14]

Freestanding ambulatory surgical centers have expanded both in number and in total procedures performed. The statistics show that 800 surgical centers performed 1.5 million procedures in 1980. The projected growth in 1990 is 1200 facilities performing 3 million procedures.[11]

Freestanding facilities will continue to grow in the 1990s because of several factors. First, technology is increasingly sophisticated and can be safely performed in a freestanding center. Diagnostic imaging services have been added to the freestanding center's system. These centers, along with physician offices, presently provide more than 20% of all imaging procedures.

Payment for outpatient delivery is still present as a less expensive setting than the acute care arena that once was the only alternative. The Health Care Financing Administration (HCFA) has increased the number of reimbursed procedures from 450 in 1982 to more than 1500 today.[11]

Private third-party reimbursers have followed HCFA's lead by encouraging patients to elect outpatient surgery to decrease costs. As a result freestanding outpatient facilities now vie with hospitals for those reimbursement dollars.

Physician Office-Based Ambulatory Care

Another player in the ambulatory care business is the physician office. For many years physicians have held the market on outpatient services as primary providers of ambulatory services. As the result of increased competition and restrictive reimbursement, group practices are occurring. The physicians join together to pool resources and patients so that volume allows high-technology acquisition. The American Medical Association states that group practices have grown 63% since 1980.[2] Hospitals have sought joint ventures with physicians to defray the competition that office-based ambulatory care provides.

Physician office ambulatory care has an advantage in that the physician sees the patient at the point of entry into the delivery system and controls the order and delivery of those procedures. Services typically associated with the physician office based ambulatory area are diagnostic imaging, physical therapy and rehabilitation, cardiovascular diagnostic services, sports medicine, and outpatient surgery. The survival of the office-based service will depend on the physicians' ability to procure state-of-the-art technology.

❖ HEALTH CARE SERVICES AVAILABLE IN THE AMBULATORY CARE SETTING

The growth of ambulatory care acceptance as an appropriate setting for health care delivery is extensive. So many services and procedures once considered unsafe and performed only in acute care now have shifted to ambulatory care. This section addresses the many options in ambulatory care.

Outpatient Surgery

Of all these services, outpatient surgery has changed and grown the most. Ambulatory surgery allows both easy access and elimination of the cost of a hospital stay. In all areas of the United States, hospitals are using the outpatient setting for at least 40% of their surgeries. In New England areas, up to 49% of surgeries are performed on an outpatient basis.[11] Although freestanding centers have increased dramatically, hospitals still hold 85% to 95% of the surgery market.[10] The most common procedures completed on an outpatient basis are cataract with lens insertion, dilatation and curettage, tonsillectomy, myringotomy, tubal ligation, arthroscopy, and erosion of skin lesions.

A major legislative incentive, the federal Omnibus Budget Reconciliation Act of 1987, has affected the growth of outpatient surgery. This promotes prospective payment for outpatient services for Medicare patients. Reimbursement is based on a blend of what HCFA would pay a freestanding surgical center and a reasonable customary rate of the hospital. A part of this legislation is defining exactly what *surgery* is, to include incision or excision, amputation, repair, suture, destruction, introduction, or manipulation. With this broad definition, procedures such as endoscopic and eye examinations or bronchoscopy and larynscopy are covered.

Another piece of this Act is the use of HCFA's common procedural coding system that must be used for outpatient procedures. This is unlike the commonly used ICD-9 coding system used in acute care settings for determining DRG payments. The provider must pay close attention to accurate coding and have the technology to accommodate this if accurate payment is to occur. This is especially important because Medicare patient claims currently make up about 20% of the total outpatient charges.[11]

Emergency Services

Emergency services are a major provider of ambulatory care. The amount and type of services provided in this setting are directly related to the availability of other organized outpatient and ambulatory care services available. Hospitals still consider the emergency department as a part of inpatient delivery for several reasons. As much as 30% of inpatient admissions go through the emergency department.[9] This area also consumes a large volume of ancillary and diagnostic resources.

In the past decade hospital emergency departments have experienced a 10% to 30% decline in usage.[10] This has been attributed to more freestanding urgent care centers with easy access and available hours, as well as discouragement by HMOs, PPOs, and insurers to use this setting for primary care. This decline has resulted in reassessment of hospital charges to differentiate between emergency and nonemergency. With better access and more reasonable charges coupled with comprehensive acute care services being available as needed, hospitals have begun to recapture this market. Some critics still contend that despite this return as many as 70% of the services provided in emergency rooms could be provided in a less costly outpatient setting.[11]

High-Technology Diagnostic Imaging and Radiology

Improved technology such as magnetic resonance imaging (MRI) and computerized tomography (CT) has changed the way health care treatments are provided in this country. Actual treatment modalities such as lithotripsy, which uses shock waves to break up kidney or gall stones, have made outpatient care a high technology industry.

Such services may be provided in the outpatient setting or in a mobile unit, providing access to areas underserved by such costly technology. Reimbursement is not keeping step with the costs as these services are receiving only modest reimbursement. Because of the costs for high technology and the lower reimbursement, many facilities are purchasing equipment together for multihospital use.

Clinical Laboratory Ambulatory Services

Outpatient laboratory testing is a very competitive area in ambulatory care delivery. At present approximately 50% to 57% of the laboratory needs are provided through hospital services with 15% to 20% occurring in independent laboratories. The remaining 15% to 20% takes place in physician offices. The predicted rate of increase is 5% annually, with physician office groups, in which most growth has come, growing about 16%.[5]

In the future more laboratory tests will be done at home, with kits already available to the public. Hospitals will have to become extremely cost efficient and may choose joint ventures with physician groups. Reimbursement for these services continues to be scrutinized. The laboratory, an area that once generated 12% of hospital funds, now costs those same hospitals dollars.[5]

Cancer Care Services

Current statistics show that approximately 30% of the U.S. population will develop cancer. This disease accounts for 10% of total disease costs in this country.[12] Hospitals have responded by developing outpatient cancer services. In fact, in a 1988 survey performed by the Ambulatory Care and Health Promotion of the American Hospital Association, 32% have done just that.[11]

This survey also pointed out the fragmentation of this ambulatory care service in the hospital arena. A comprehensive outpatient cancer care program would include multidisciplinary treatment assessment with full radiation capabilities, tumor registry, support services, and chemotherapy. Fragmentation and reimbursement incentives have produced competitors such as freestanding cancer centers and physician office practices. Medicare alone pays for 43% of the cancer outpatient services.[11] Certain changes may affect this niche, such as a decrease in reimbursement and prospective payment incentives in the 1990s.

Cardiovascular Ambulatory Services

With 65 million Americans having cardiovascular disease, this is the largest segment of the health care market. Most cardiovascular services have always been considered inpatient services, except for diagnostic procedures such as electrocardiography (ECG). Today some invasive procedures such as the cardiac catheterization can be safely performed in the outpatient setting. More and more noninvasive procedures such as vascular imaging are being developed to encourage the shift of cardiovascular diagnosis and treatment to the ambulatory care setting.

Few freestanding cardiovascular outpatient centers have developed because of prohibition by the states. If care is performed away from the hospital ambulatory setting, the cardiovascular services are performed in a physician's office. Pilot projects that are currently underway will give data to support or negate the usefulness and costs of ambulatory cardiovascular services. In fact mobile units may be the answer to access in rural and underserved areas.

Ambulatory Rehabilitation Services

Rehabilitation services, which have experienced growth in the past decade, can be delivered in various settings including the hospital inpatient setting, freestanding rehabilitation center, home care, and outpatient setting. Again the multidisciplinary approach is most effective in controlling costs and providing a positive outcome.

During the 1990s one can expect the continued expansion of medical rehabilitation services. Specific service areas include cardiac rehabilitation, pediatric rehabilitation, worker and industrial rehabilitation, and head injury rehabilitation. With prospective payment looming on the horizon most programs will be ambulatory, with only the sickest patients remaining in the hospital. Competition will be aggressive as providers develop ambulatory services to meet this health care market need.

Other Ambulatory Services

Other services also will move to ambulatory care. Outpatient clinics will offer special services in diabetes, arthritis, allergies, pain management, sleep disorders, and digestive disorders. Other ambulatory services for the 1990s are women's health, sports medicine, occupational and industrial medicine, health promotion activities, and behavioral medicine.

Home care and hospice services are outpatient areas that continue to expand. It is clear that the health care industry has just begun to effectively use the ambulatory care delivery system in the United States.

❖ AMBULATORY CARE: UNIQUE ISSUES

Although ambulatory care is in an infancy stage as a delivery system, it is viewed as a profitable and important health care niche. As the gross national product rises to 15% by the year 2000, ambulatory care, like all other settings, must confront unique challenges.[13]

Reimbursement

Medicare payments for outpatient services have had a significant growth rate. The federal government is now looking at this payment system. The reform of Medicare B will force providers to increase efficiency and productivity in the outpatient arena.

Private insurers continue to initiate cost containment programs. Two thirds of all health care presently is funded through insurance companies offered by employers.[6] Some employers are building in incentives for employees to use ambulatory or outpatient services to decrease costs. More than 90% of these companies require a second opinion for surgical cases.[6] The copayments are increasing, with shared health risks between the employer and employee. *Managed care* programs are including outpatient services as a key part of the health care delivery system.

Productivity Evaluations

As outpatient departments deliver a variety of services and include a multidisciplinary team approach, ambulatory care can become labor intensive. With reimbursement margins shrinking with prospective payment, productivity evaluations will become increasingly crucial to ambulatory service viability.

Hospitals must develop measures to monitor utilization of resources. Procedures must be clinically justified. Management must be creative and responsive to ensure maximum productivity and operational effectiveness.

Information Management Systems

Another key challenge to ambulatory care is information management systems. As previously stated, coding is crucial to payment. The current procedural terminology (CPT-4) is the most prevalent system for outpatient coding. Making a change from the traditional ICD-9 coding programs is labor intensive because coders must learn to use another language. Also there are still few experienced vendors for automated ambulatory care management because of the constant change of the environment. Much ambulatory care data management is still a manual process.

Quality in Ambulatory Care

As with all health care settings, quality of patient services and outcomes is being scrutinized. Certain aspects of outpatient care complicate the measurement and documentation of outpatient quality care. These include the volume of patients through the various settings, the assessment of outcomes with a mobile target population, less than optimal medical record functions, and subjective assessments of factors affecting patient outcomes.

The American Hospital Association has an organization, The Quality Assurance Committee of the Society for Ambulatory Care Professionals, dedicated to this function. This group asserts that ambulatory care must be of equal quality as inpatient hospital care. Certain attributes are defined to measure ambulatory care quality, which are[11] (1) effectiveness of the care delivered and technical competency, (2) the acceptability of the outpatient service, (3) availability/access to the service, (4) continuity of care, and (5) the *value-added* concept.

❖ INTEGRATED QUALITY MANAGEMENT IN THE AMBULATORY CARE SETTING

Regardless of the setting for ambulatory care, nursing practice plays a major role. Nurses provide direct and indirect care of patients in these outpatient settings, with less control over the outcomes of their practice. It is of grave importance that ambulatory care nurses understand and integrate quality management (QM) into their daily practice.

Outpatient Surgery

A patient enters the ambulatory care setting as an outpatient short-stay surgery patient. The nurse must first determine if this is the appropriate setting to treat this patient, which is an example of *utilization management*. If the surgery is appropriate to the setting, the nurse assesses the patient's ability to have the surgery in this setting. An example is the uncomplicated cataract surgery routinely performed in the outpatient surgery center. If the patient happens to be an elderly female with severe arrhythmias and prominent dehydration after having pneumonia, the nurse would question the appropriateness of this setting. The nurse has demonstrated *utilization management, risk management, safety,* and *infection control*.

A key aspect of care in the outpatient surgery nursing practice is pain management and comfort measures. This is an appropriate area to monitor and evaluate for any change in postoperative status because of pain or nausea and vomiting. This aspect of care has direct implications for nursing measures that can produce a better patient outcome.

Another QA indicator in ambulatory surgery is patient education. The ambulatory nurse must use the short time available to provide presurgery and postsurgery patient education. This must be accomplished in such a way as to decrease the patient's chance of an adverse outcome once discharged to the home setting. In some patients a home visit by a home care nurse is appropriate and can decrease the chance of an adverse outcome after surgery. Patient education is a QA indicator that can minimize inappropriate readmission to the acute care setting through patient and/or care giver understanding of what to expect after surgery and how to handle any complications.

Another very important part of quality management in the ambulatory surgery patient is patient satisfaction. The patient is the best judge of whether the nursing care received was helpful and useful. A formal follow-up program of discharged patients within a 24 to 48 hour postoperative time frame will show the patient that the nurse cares about the patient even after discharge. This is also a good *risk management* tool to check on any complication or patient complaints that may need discussing. It addresses *utilization management* because it can decrease admission to an acute care setting if the patient needs referral to an appropriate area for follow-up such as home care.

Outpatient Surgery Generic Quality Screens

Documentation of patient care in the medical record is extremely important and part of the role of the professional nurse. The Peer Review Organization (PRO) reviews the outpatient surgery chart with definite quality screens.[7] The nurse should be aware of these and build quality monitors around these screens.

The first screen is adequacy of preoperative assessment, including a timely history and physical examination by the physician, with results in the chart. The operative note must include information about the operative site. Another area in this assessment is the laboratory tests, ECG, and x-ray films reviewed before surgery. Vital signs must be taken. Any abnormal results must be corrected or addressed in the record if they are unresolved. The operative record is also examined for deviations in vital signs and timely interventions.

Issues related to postoperative care are reviewed in these screens. The screens look at vital signs, serious life-threatening complications, major adverse drug reactions, and change in a patient's mental status. Other screens that relate directly to the nurse are (1) documentation of appropriate discharge plan with provisions for follow-up care and (2) adequate patient education.

The ambulatory care surgery nurse has many opportunities to affect the quality and appropriateness of care in that setting. This nurse must examine the scope of practice unique to that area and define the various areas for QM monitoring and evaluation.

Outpatient Clinic

Professional nurses are traditionally the primary care givers of many patients in the outpatient clinic setting. In fact many clinic settings are managed by the nurse clinician who has a master's degree. Clinic nurses can work with patients from all areas of health care including pediatrics, cardiology, pulmonary, oncology, urology, ophthalmology, neurology, and general medicine. Regardless of the particular type of patient seen, the professional nurse has several quality management concerns.

Health teaching must be done, and it must be ongoing to enhance the patient health care outcome. Patients must have treatments and procedures explained and demonstrate understanding. Patient compliance is a desired outcome but may not always occur. The nurse must have excellent interpersonal skills to work with patients who are slow to comply with prescribed therapies.

Hospital Outpatient Department Generic Quality Screens

As previously discussed outpatient clinic care is often part of the hospital delivery systems. The PRO generic quality screens again are aimed at adequate assessment to include medical, physical, psychologic, and social conditions of the patient. Another part is a *utilization management* issue: is the outpatient department the appropriate setting for this patient?

The second screen is appropriate and timely interventions. The PRO reviews the chart for appropriate diagnosis and therapeutic services that are provided and determines if they are based on the assessment of the patient needs. The record must address any abnormal results of diagnostic services. The chart must reflect reassessment of patient needs and appropriate referral to other disciplines delineated as necessary. This outpatient setting is an area in which interdisciplinary collaboration on quality management concerns can make a difference in patient care outcomes. In fact the third screen addresses specialty therapy assessments and the patient's compliance with the plan.

The fourth screen reviews a major piece of nursing process and practice. It looks for documentation of assessment of the patient's educational needs with development of patient plan of care. The evaluation process of this plan must also be documented along with the monitoring of patient compliance to the prescribed health care plan. Patient education must always be part of the outpatient nurse's QA plan.

The PRO reviews all records if a patient is admitted to the hospital and dies within 48 hours. Other critical screens include serious, life-threatening complications as a result of inadequate care, severe adverse reaction to a medication or a medication error, unstable vital signs, purulent or bloody drainage from a wound, and any infection following a dressing change or invasive procedure. *Risk management, safety,* and *infection control* aspects of quality management come into focus with these screens.

Another nursing QA indicator might be the documented plan for discharge and follow-up care at discharge. Discharge planning is part of nursing process and practice. The PRO looks for this in the outpatient setting just as in the acute setting.

The generic quality screens are generally applied by the PRO nurse. In the outpatient setting the reviewer is asked to state if he or she sees any trend or pattern of events that resulted in adverse outcomes that need to be investigated. If so the record is reviewed further by the PRO physician.

Outpatient Invasive Procedure Documentation

The PRO has suggestions for documenting the care of the patient who has an invasive procedure in any ambulatory setting, whether it be outpatient surgery or the gastrointestinal laboratory. The suggestions include examination of the patient immediately before the procedure to determine any **risk** for anesthesia or adverse outcome. A history and physical must be present. Also one should document known allergies, current medications and dosages, as well as a mental assessment and rationale for the planned procedure.

Actual reports from the laboratory, ECG, or x-ray departments must be present, along with vital signs taken before the procedure. Again any abnormal results from diagnostic tests or vital signs must be explained completely in the record if they remain unresolved. Vital signs must be taken before, during, and after the procedure regardless of the anesthesia used. Abnormal values must be identified with the timely interventions.

Before patient discharge the physician must evaluate and document proper recovery from anesthesia. The patient must have a discharge plan that reflects the appropriate transition in care and identifies any additional resources needed, such as follow-up care. Again adequate education must be documented as a major quality indicator.

QM Clinical Indicators in Ambulatory Care Services

Sometimes it helps to review sample indicators to clarify possible QM indicators appropriate for ambulatory care. Some *risk* outcome indicators are the following[3]:
1. Wrong patient for the procedure/treatment
2. Patient injury/visitor injury

3. Patient leaves AMA/refuses treatment
4. Unexpected death/code
5. Failure to regain consciousness after surgery
6. Unexpected medication/transfusion reaction other than mild rash or itching
7. Return to surgery for removal of retained foreign body (iatrogenic)

Some outcome indicators that are appropriate for administrative review of the *process* used in ambulatory care could be the following[3]:

1. Equipment malfunctions or is unavailable
2. Specimen loss
3. Correct sponge, needle, instrument, or tooth count
4. Loss or damage to personal articles

Quality outcome indicators in an ambulatory care setting might include the following:

1. Medication/transfusion error requiring intervention (risk management/safety)
2. Aspiration (risk management/safety/infection control)
3. Unplanned return to surgery or acute care admission (utilization management/risk management)
4. Laceration or perforation of body part or organ during an invasive procedure (risk management/safety/utilization management)
5. Surgery canceled after patient in operating room (utilization management)

Using Indicators for Quality Assessment and Improvement

All above indicators can be used to identify areas needing quality assessment and improvement. For example, in indicator three, unplanned return to surgery or acute care admission would be appropriate for quality assessment and improvement. If a patient has an acute care admission following ambulatory surgery, the nurse might review the ambulatory care preoperative, the operative, and postoperative records. This would allow examination for any possible problem that could be improved to prevent the adverse outcome of *admission*. Questions one might assess are the following:

1. Was the patient's preoperative assessment effective? Were there any gaps? Were all needed disciplines included in the plan?
2. Was the appropriateness for ambulatory surgery evaluated accurately? Were there unforeseen circumstances that would have im-

proved the outcome had they been known by the ambulatory care team before surgery?
3. Were the possible risk and safety factors for ambulatory surgery assessed proactively?
4. Was patient/family education provided before surgery in an appropriate way with reverbalizing of care taught? Was this process begun early enough to allow for proper learning? Were questions encouraged?
5. Did preoperative assessment include infection control concerns when indicated?

One way to answer these questions is to use a crossfunctional or interdisciplinary case conference to review all data. This team may become a *quality improvement team* to identify all possible opportunities for improvements in the ambulatory care process. In this way one case study by this team can improve patient care and minimize another similar adverse outcome. Any information from the process would be communicated to everyone involved in the process. Assessing the quality from many different points can improve the process and improve patient care outcomes.

❖ NATIONAL DEMONSTRATION PROJECT ON QUALITY IMPROVEMENT IN HEALTH CARE (NDP): AN EXAMPLE IN AMBULATORY CARE

The Park Nicollet Center team chose ambulatory care as its focus in developing a quality improvement process for review.[4] The team decided to assess the satisfaction of its external customers. Team members came up with 23 different "likely causes" and sent surveys to more than 7000 patients, seeking their review.

The team compiled the results by frequency, using a pareto diagram. Interesting results were discovered. Six of the 23 "likely causes" were not cited by any of the patients. Obviously, had the team begun the process by addressing these six, valuable time would have been wasted and no positive change would have resulted.

The most common problem from the survey was "telephone access"—difficulty getting to a physician and having to wait for an excessive time. This leading cause was suspected by the administration, but no solution was apparent. The team developed the following goal: "to improve the entire process of obtaining the medical record information and/or appointment by telephone in the family practice section of the medical center."

As the study continued, it became apparent that the time when telephone access peaked was when two receptionists were called to a training meeting. This is what is known as a *special cause variant* because the problem was not with process itself but with a particular time or reason in the process. Management changed the time of the training meeting from the business hours.

Another problem discovered in the study was that the receptionist answered the call within 15 seconds while the medical information nurse answered in 60 to 90 seconds. The team focused efforts on improving process capability of the medical information nurse.

The quality improvement team assessed and improved the satisfaction of patients in the ambulatory care area. This was accomplished by data collection, displays using visual tools such as the pareto diagram, and analysis. This is one example of quality assessment and improvement by the NDP in the area of ambulatory care.

❖ SUMMARY

Nursing practice transcends the varied ambulatory settings in key aspects of care. Certain important aspects of care remain consistent, such as nursing process, patient education, and discharge planning. Quality management in the ambulatory care setting also remains consistent as the nurse must integrate utilization management, quality assessment and improvement, risk management, safety, and infection control. Customer satisfaction in any setting is paramount in quality management. Although there are unique issues and challenges for the nurse practicing in the ambulatory care setting, the goal of providing appropriate care in the appropriate setting with positive patient care outcomes remains the same.

REFERENCES

1. American Hospital Association, *Hospital Statistics,* Chicago, Ill, 1984, 1988.
2. American Medical Association, *Physician characteristics and distribution in the United States,* Chicago, 1987.
3. Bassett S, Schladermundt L: *Sample clinical indicators,* Deerfield, Ill, 1989, National Association of Quality Assurance Professionals.
4. Berwick DM, Godfrey AB, Roessner J: *Curing health care: new strategies for quality improvement,* San Francisco, 1990, Jossey-Bass.

5. Biomedical Business International: *Clinical laboratory services industry,* No. 70776, Tustin, Calif, 1987.
6. *The business roundtable, health, welfare, and retirement income task force report: corporate health-care-cost management and private sector initiatives,* Indianapolis, 1987, The Business Roundtable.
7. *Generic quality screens, third scope of work,* Mid-South Foundation for Medical Care, August 1990.
8. Matson TA: *The explosive growth of ambulatory care: challenges and opportunities for hospitals,* Barrington, Ill, Nov. 28, 1986, Evangelical Health Systems, Good Shepard Hospital.
9. Matson TA: *The hospital emergency department in transition,* The Hospital Emergency Department: Returning to Financial Viability Conference, Chicago, July, 16, 1986, American Hospital Association
10. Matson TA: *Rethinking the delivery of ambulatory care: hospital-based versus freestanding alternatives,* Penetrating the Alternative Site Market Place Conference, San Francisco, Sept. 15, 1987, Biomedical Business International.
11. Matson TA, editor: *Restructuring for ambulatory care: a guide to reorganization.* Division of ambulatory care and promotion, 1990, American Hospital Publishing.
12. Nathanson SN, Lerman D: *Outpatient cancer centers: implementation and management,* Chicago, 1988, American Hospital Publishing.
13. National health expenditures, 1987, *Health Care Review,* Winter, 1988.
14. SMG marketing group, *Freestanding ambulatory care center report and directory,* Chicago, June 1987.

CHAPTER

13

❖

Quality Management in Home Health Care

❖ EVOLUTION AND INFLUENCES ON HOME HEALTH CARE NURSING

Home health care can be traced to the early Christian Church. It is historically evident that people made home visits to provide health care. Later, religious orders such as the Sisters of Charity founded by St. Vincent De Paul of France began making home visits to provide health care. The oldest established home nursing service in the United States is the Ladies Benevolent Society in South Carolina, which was established in 1813.

Florence Nightingale endorsed the idea of home nursing when the administrators of the school where she was trained conceived the idea of extending nursing services provided in the hospital to the sick in their homes. In 1859 Nightingale participated in the creation of the first district public health nursing association in England.

Community health nursing developed in the United States as a unique area of practice, and in 1877 the first trained nurses were employed by the Women's Branch of the New York City Mission to provide home nursing services. In the following years district nursing associations were established in various cities, with some instituting fees for service. The concept of community health supervisor and the role as educator, as well as caretaker of the sick, also were established.

As community nursing grew, the need for standardization of community nursing practice was recognized. In response, in 1911 a committee of the

American Nurses Association and the Society for Superintendents of Training Schools for Nurses met to address the need. The result of this collaboration was the formation of the National Organization for Public Health Nursing, whose objectives were to provide stimulation and standardization of public health nursing.

In 1964 the American Nurses Association (ANA) defined the public health nurse as a graduate of a baccalaureate program in nursing in response to the recognition of the uniqueness and skills required to provide community health nursing. The Child Health Act of 1967 and the Health Maintenance Organization Act of 1973 recommended the use of nurses in an extended role. The report, entitled "An Abstract for Nursing," which was a joint effort of the American Nurses Association and the National League for Nursing and published in 1970, recognized community health as an important field of care. The groups divided patient care into two basic areas: episodic care relating to restorative and curative care for the sick and distributive care that is preventive in nature.

Home health nursing, an original component of community health nursing, evolved in the United States as a unique nursing practice innovation. Home health care integrates the principles and practices of nursing, performing both preventive and curative services. In the beginning of the twentieth century most home health nursing was provided by visiting nurse associations and nursing departments of city or county health departments.

Growth in home health care was a result of the expanded role of the nurse, and further expansion occurred when Medicare and Medicaid were created, which became major sources of third-party payment for home health care services. Further growth occurred when PPS introduced cost containment, and decreased lengths of stay in the hospital became evident. Since the inception of home health care, services have continued to diversify; yet one constant has remained, namely, nursing as the organizer, planner, and provider of the majority of care.

Home health care is the single major provider of care to the chronically ill, frail, and elderly. Home health care is an alternative to costly institutional care, giving the elderly an opportunity to stay at home and receive care. In 1981 the National Association for Home Care estimated that 4 million people in the United States used home care services, and by 1995 projections are that $14.2 billion will be spent on home health care.

The first hospital-based home health care agency was established at Montefiore Hospital in New York in the early 1940s. Present-day agencies provide a wide variety of services in various combinations. Services of all types are initiated by order of a physician and are under his or her supervision. Patients treated by contemporary agencies vary from pediatric to the elderly.

❖ HIGH TECHNOLOGY AND HOME HEALTH CARE CHALLENGE

In the pretechnology era health care was often provided in the home. It was not uncommon for a physician to make home visits and have office hours. For several decades the major source of health care was the acute care institution and a generation of physicians who managed the high technology care. Today we are reverting in some ways to the pretechnology era but now with technology that can be used in homes.

Chemotherapeutic drugs and pain control via pumps are now available in the home setting. Continuing technology facilitates safe and cost-effective infusion therapies such as antibiotics. Increased sophistication and simplification of techniques exist for remote monitoring of patients, equipment, and systems. Services of all types and for all ages will be delivered at home.

Demographic, technologic, and economic trends will continue to affect how care is delivered. Home health care nurses will continue to be challenged in dealing with the changing population composition, the increasing numbers of elderly, and ever-changing resource availability, in addition to increasing technology.

Nursing roles will continue to evolve in home health care, with health promotion and prevention of illness as major components. Increased mobility of the population and instability of the family will contribute to greater stress in an era in which support systems may be negligible. Nurses will need to be alert to all types of health problems and assist patients in the development of alternative support systems and learning problem solving skills.

❖ HOSPICE MOVEMENT IN THE UNITED STATES

The evolution of home health care hospice programs has become more notable in recent years. The major goal of a hospice is symptom relief and preparation for death. Hospices that are nonresidential strive to help the patient die at home, if he or she wishes, as opposed to an institutional setting. Hospice patients are encouraged to discuss their feelings regarding death and to put their affairs in order. The hospice affords the patient the opportunity to bid farewell to loved ones, and the patient's family is also the recipient of the hospice care.

For patients a hospice provides a sense of control over some aspects of the dying patient's life. Patients receive loving care and support of their decision to die without extraordinary means to prolong life. Patients receive pain relief to the extent possible and the support of the nurse throughout the dying process. The hospice nurse is a facilitator of efforts of the patient to put his or her affairs in order and bid farewell to family and friends.

The family of the hospice patient receives guidance, as well as emotional support, in the care of the patient. Families of the hospice patient also receive grief support after the death of their loved one; therefore the care and support does not end with the death of the patient. The family is also supported to accept the wishes of the hospice patient regarding care and final arrangements such as the funeral and related matters. Many private insurers have joined Medicare in the endorsement of hospices and the provision for payment for hospice services. Often hospice care is the most cost-efficient care alternative, especially when the patient chooses to die at home. Because the care focuses on palliative and pain control, the cost of the care is often greatly reduced, even if the patient requires continuous nursing care in the home for a period of time.

❖ HMO/PPO USE OF HOME HEALTH CARE

Health Maintenance Organizations (HMOs) and Preferred Provider Organizations (PPOs) have a significant share of the population as enrollees, and that is expected to continue to rise. Because HMOs provide health care services themselves to control cost and resource utilization, they limit the use of home health care agencies to those that offer services at a reduced cost. Unlike HMOs, PPOs do not provide the services themselves but act as brokers for the purchase of discounted health services. Patients are given economic incentives to use certain providers within the approved group as specified by the PPO.

❖ TYPES OF HOME HEALTH CARE AGENCIES

Official health agencies are the oldest type of home health care providers and are funded through state and local taxes. Generally these agencies are a division of a state or local health department.

Voluntary home health organizations are financed through groups such as heart associations, cancer societies, and third-party payors and do not receive tax dollars. Historically, voluntary organizations have depended primarily on the nurse for service delivery, and today most have comprehensive services, with varied disciplines providing care.

Private home health agencies may be nonprofit or proprietary, which are owned by an individual or corporation. Private agencies may not participate in Medicare or Medicaid, and funding comes from third-party payors.

Hospital-based home health agencies may be nonprofit or proprietary and receive funds from Medicare, Medicaid and third-party payors. Hospital-based programs generally provide an array of services and cite continuity of care as the major advantage of these agencies.

❖ HOME HEALTH CARE AND FISCAL INTERMEDIARY RELATIONSHIP

Fiscal intermediaries (FIs) are public or private groups designated by the federal government to perform the following:
1. Process claims for Medicare patients
2. Monitor services that are delivered to federal health insurance clients for appropriateness
3. Act as a consultant to providers regarding services covered under federal insurance

❖ CONTINUOUS QUALITY IMPROVEMENT IN HOME HEALTH CARE

CQI implementation in home health care is a never-ending cycle of improvement based on needs defined by the customers. Federal, state, and fiscal intermediaries give guidelines for what they consider appropriate services, documentation, and other matters. Standardized forms such as those required for submission of bills to the FI serve as a national source of information regarding services provided to clients. Adherence to guidelines provided by regulatory bodies is just one step in the delivery of quality patient care. Because the care given in home health is focused on nursing, nurses have an enormous opportunity to affect the quality of care as a major system of care in an environment less controlled than the acute care setting. The lack of a controlled environment and diversity of services pose special challenges to continuous quality improvement efforts, particularly because care is not provided in a central location.

❖ QUALITY ASSESSMENT IN HOME HEALTH CARE

Quality assessment in home health care has evolved over time. Home health care has unique problems related to quality assessment because of the uncontrolled environment. Maintenance of a person in his or her own home involves support of a patient's health and functional abilities yet preservation of his or her personal lifestyle. Monitoring and evaluation activities are more difficult in home health care because there are fewer controls than there are in the acute care setting. Early standards for home health care quality assessment focused more on the education of the nurses who provided home care.

Before 1965 the major emphasis regarding quality assessment in home care was the supervision of nurses in the field, the annual evaluation of agency functioning, the collection of statistical data on patients and patient care to project future needs, and nursing education requirements. Quality assessment activities today are often dictated by the regulations established by state, local, and federal government. Medicare introduced home health care coverage when it was created in 1965. There was no standardized quality assessment process, but the legislation included criteria for eligibility of the patient and conditions of participation for agencies who were billing Medicare or accepting Medicare patients.

In 1966 the American Nurses Association created divisions of practice that established standards of care in the specialty areas of nursing. The Community Health Standard was introduced in 1973 and later revised in 1986. The National League for Nursing has an accreditation program for community health and home health care agencies. Joint Commission standards for home health care became effective in June 1988.

Quality assessment in home health care has several general approaches. These efforts focus on agency structure and licensure and certification of health providers. Specific approaches to quality assessment are related to review mechanisms to monitor processes and outcomes. State, federal, and local agencies often dictate quality assessment requirements in their regulations. In an effort to control cost and determine agency compliance to regulation, different types of audits are performed. External reviews are performed by FIs, state licensing or Medicare certification reviewers, or HCFA regional surveyors. FIs review use and cost of services through what is called compliance or fiscal audits. State licensure surveyors determine whether an agency complies with requirements for Medicare conditions of participation by focusing on evidence that agencies perform quality assessment audits. Medicare compliance audits involve review of client records for accuracy of documentation and the medical need for care.

Regulatory and quality requirements are not met when unqualified staff members provide care, supervision is lacking, documentation is poor, or services are overutilized. Agency regulations require that professional and medical staff review plan of care at least every 60 days for appropriateness and continued care. A clinical record review must be performed quarterly on a percentage of open and closed cases. An advisory committee, composed of agency and nonagency professionals and consumers, must review policies and procedures periodically. The advisory committee must review the home health care agency program annually.

❖ RISK MANAGEMENT IN HOME HEALTH CARE

In the 1970s and 1980s litigation against hospitals and physicians rose dramatically. Generally home health care agencies did not experience the same increase. Despite this fact several risks are inherent in the home health care industry, and as growth and diversification of services continue, the risk factors will also increase. Risks in home health care are associated with the lack of environmental controls where the care is provided, services being provided with little supervision, and the fact that high quality outcomes are very strongly associated with the patient's or care giver's knowledge, ability, and compliance with the plan of care.

The home health care agency is labor intensive, requiring personnel with varied credentials, training, and expertise. Hiring of staff from a risk management perspective requires devising specific criteria and expectations to decrease the risk of litigation. This can best be accomplished through very detailed job descriptions, skill level assessments, and performance evaluations.

Staff members will need ongoing continuing education, particularly when new technology is introduced. The staff must be able to communicate and teach the new information to assist patients and care givers in understanding use and techniques. The timeliness of the services provided and after-hours coverage are risk management concerns, as is insurance coverage of company vehicles. Inclement weather also poses serious problems related to staff safety, as well as the concerns over compromising care to patients. Documentation is crucial, just as in inpatient settings. Detailed, well-maintained records are the first line of defense in litigation, and adequate professional insurance is a must.

The bond that traditionally occurs in the home health care setting between the provider, the patient, and the family is unique and often an asset in the prevention of legal problems. Confidence in the care giver is the strongest asset any agency can possess. Clear, concise admission and discharge criteria facilitate a basic understanding of the care the agency can and cannot provide. The screening of referrals for appropriateness for admission is critical. Accepting a patient whose care is beyond the scope of the services provided by the agency poses a risk to the agency and endangers the health of that patient. After acceptance of an individual for care, consistent verbal and written communication is essential. All staff should be carefully screened and supervised closely to avoid problems with patient abuse and neglect. Patients should feel comfortable to discuss their concerns with agency administration or call appropriate authorities. Clear protocols for the administration of drugs and use of equipment including backup systems will aid the agency in avoiding legal problems. In an emergency situation the agency staff should stay with the patient until further assistance arrives or the patient knows what the proper procedure is. Proper instruction is without question the key issue in preventing problems.

Actual or perceived expectations of the patient or care giver can pose risk management concerns in the home environment. Therefore clear and thorough explanations of treatment and planning, as well as emphasis on patient rights and responsibilities, should be given during admission. For example, the care givers may believe that the nurse will visit four times a day to administer intravenous antibiotics, but in reality the nurse is going to provide the first few doses with the intent to teach the care giver or patient to administer the medication.

Patient/care giver satisfaction is subjective and reflects personal preferences, as well as expectations. Personal preference is reflected in the dimension of satisfaction, including the availability of care, provider competence, communication of the provider, and personal qualities of the provider. The patient's personality may clash with that of the provider, or there may be a problem with the care provider and home care giver that diminishes the potential for positive interchange, thus decreasing the perceived quality of care, which poses potential risks.

❖ HOME HEALTH CARE AND INFECTION CONTROL

The basic elements of infection control, such as proper handwashing techniques, disposal of needles, and so on, apply in the home health care setting just as in any other. Inherent problems with infection control exist because the home environment can be controlled less than an institutional setting. Another contributor to the spread of infectious disease is that the care giver in the home will provide the majority of the care. The nursing role is crucial in teaching aseptic principles. The patient or care giver may not understand how cross-contamination can occur when touching a draining wound or dressings from a draining wound and then diapering an infant in the home, or how important good nutrition and cleanliness are to wound healing.

Other issues in infection control relate to the availability of resources such as inside plumbing and running water. The aptitude of the care giver also plays a role in the quality of the care, as well as the interest of the support persons for the patient. All of the issues should be assessed by the nurse and documented. Information and problems that are identified should be reported to the patient's physician, documented in the record, and reported to the administrative arm of the agency. Guidelines for care and infection control practices are provided by various state and local agencies and accrediting agencies such as the Joint Commission and the individual state licensure bodies.

❖ HOME HEALTH CARE AND UTILIZATION MANAGEMENT

Medicare has established utilization standards for home health care. These standards establish guidelines for appropriateness of admission and continued care in home health. Individual states are allowed to control state funding for home health care. Although states are regulated to some extent by the federal government, they have greater autonomy to administer their funds such as Medicaid. Generally Medicare funds for home health cannot be used for maintenance care of a patient or for prevention.

Patients must be assessed from the referral point if they are appropriate for the level of care that the home health care agency provides, and after admission there must be continual assessment if the patient meets the criteria for continued service by home health care as established under guidelines. Guidelines include agency admission, continued care, or discharge criteria, and state, federal, and accrediting body standards. During the period when a patient is receiving home health care there must also be continual assessment by the providers of the care concerning whether the patient continues to meet criteria for continued care, for inpatient acute care, or long-term care admission, or if the patient is appropriate for discharge. For example, patients who are not homebound or who are well enough to be out of the home without great assistance are not appropriate for home health care services. Agencies that do not have adequate staff to render care to patients on ventilators should not accept ventilator patients for admission.

Home health care can be tremendously important in aiding acute care facilities in addressing their utilization issues. Those patients no longer appropriate for inpatient admission can often receive the level of care by using home health, which provides benefits to both the patient and the institution. The patient can receive the care needed, and the institution can control cost, as well as meet the guidelines established by the Peer Review Organization (PRO) for inpatient admission or continued stay. Home health care can also be an alternative for postoperative patients from ambulatory settings as opposed to an inpatient admission.

❖ FUTURE HOME HEALTH CARE

For centuries care has been delivered in the homes of patients. For many years care of the sick was provided by family members with the help of visiting nurses and visiting physicians. Technology initiated a trend toward inpatient care, and a new breed of physician educated and trained to treat patients with this new technology emerged. The creation of Medicare and Medicaid initiated a huge market for this new technology, and after a brief period of time recognition that the cost of unlimited care for increasing numbers of people could not be supported by the federal government.

Medicare and Medicaid reimbursement for home health care caused tremendous growth. The introduction of PPOs and DRGs further expanded the market because patients were discharged sooner and often needed some level of nonacute care.

Home health care is seen as a cost-effective means of delivering care. Technology for use in the home setting is also increasing, creating more opportunities for even the very ill to remain at home. Services are continuing to expand and are expected to continue to grow.

❖ IMPLICATIONS FOR NURSING

Although home health care is the oldest form of ambulatory care, only in recent years has there been increased growth. Many services can be provided in the home setting, and greater technology is available for home use.

Increased growth and diversified services will require the skills of many nurses. These factors will give nurses a variety of specialty areas in which to practice in the home health care field. The independence of the practice and lack of environmental controls will challenge the nurse to use his or her skills and creative abilities in planning and providing care. Home health care nurses will need good communication skills and interviewing techniques. Nurses providing home health care will need to be broad-based in knowledge of diagnoses, treatments, and disease processes. Nurses will coordinate care and must be able to collaborate with other disciplines to provide the best care possible.

❖ SUMMARY

People are living longer and are affected by more chronic illnesses requiring medical intervention during their life span. Technologic advances, changes in the reimbursement structure, and greater governmental control over who may be admitted to acute care and how long they may stay have forced the use of home health care as an alternative means of care that is often more cost effective.

Home health care hospice agencies have proved beneficial to patients and families and are often more cost effective. Referral sources range from the physician, nurse, and patient to Health Maintenance Organizations and Preferred Provider Organizations looking for cost-efficient services. A wider range of services are available in the home, including high-tech services such as total parenteral nutrition and enteral nutrition. Home health care has unique issues related to infection control and risk management because the home environment is difficult to control. Quality assessment is more critical because the environment is not under the scrutiny of other settings such as acute care or ambulatory units. Home health nursing will face new challenges as diversification opens new areas of home health care services. Home health care growth is expected to continue as a means of cost containment and is a shift from inpatient care.

REFERENCES

1. Clark MJD:*Community health nursing for today and tomorrow,* Reston, Va, 1984, Reston Publishing.
2. Seddall-Stuart S:*Home health care nursing, administrative and clinical perspectives,* Rockville, Md, 1986, Aspen Publishers.
3. Bay JK, Nestman L, Bayda B: Attitudes and opinions of physicians toward a coordinated home program, *Can J Public Health* 6(74):50, 1983.
4. Boyle T: Home care contracting with Health Maintenance Organizations and Preferred Provider Organizations, *Caring,* 2, 1987.
5. Brueckner G: Implementing an effective home care risk management program, *Perspectives in Health Care Risk Management,* Fall 1989.
6. Dahlberg NLF: A perinatal center based antepartum homecare program, *JOGN,* January/February 1988.
7. Halamandaris VJ: Home care: the future of medicine, *Journal of Physicians in Home Care,* pp. 20-21, Spring 1987.
8. Harris MD: Clinical and financial outcomes in patient care in home health care agency, *J Nurs Qual Assur* 5(2):41–49, 1991.
9. Hopkins JL: Increased quality and reduced risk in the home care setting, *QRC Advisor, Managing Hospital Quality and Risk, and Cost* 3(10), 1987.
10. Hrusovsky I: High-tech home care delivery, *Journal for Physicians in Home Care,* pp. 43-51, Spring, 1987.
11. Koren MJ, Schrague H: Psychiatric home care, *Journal for Physicians in Home Care,* pp. 64-72, 1987.
12. Louden T: Hospitals eager for a larger share of growing home health market, *Modern Health Care* 14:66-68, 1984.
13. Perren JM: Chronically ill children in America; the case for home care, *Journal for Physicians in Home Care,* Spring, pp. 54–62, 1987.
14. Popovich MA: Planning the QA program for a hospital-based home health agency, *Hospital Home Health* 8:118-121, September, 1991.

CHAPTER

14

❖

Quality Management in Long-Term Care

❖ INTRODUCTION

THE phrase *the graying of America* aptly describes an increasing segment of the U.S. population. At the turn of the century, 1 in 25 people was 65 or older, 4% of the overall population. Predictions for the year 2000 are that 1 in 5 will be 65 or older. This increase in the elderly population is attributed to several factors. Birth rates fell in the nineteenth and twentieth centuries. After World War I a significant number of Europeans emigrated whose children are now 65 or older. Life expectancy has increased as a result of improved diagnosis and disease treatment and improved nutrition and standard of living.

❖ AGING, ILLNESS, AND INFLUENCING FACTORS

The aging process begins at conception. The rate of aging is very individualized but accelerates in later years. Aging encompasses physiologic, sociologic, and biologic components. As one ages, the incidence of chronic disease also increases. Heart disease, cancer, and strokes account for the major illnesses of the elderly, which in turn require frequent and longer hospital stays, rehabilitation, and long-term care units. As aging continues, the incidence of conditions requiring health care increases.

Chronic diseases have largely replaced communicable diseases as a major health problem in the United States. Chronic illness generally has a gradual onset and is a condition characterized by slow, progressive decline, requiring continual medical therapy and nursing intervention. Approximately 86% of the older adults have one or more chronic diseases.

Social trends, which include demographics, technologic advance, politics, and economics, influence health care delivery. Urbanization and increased mobility have decreased the stability of the family and available support systems. Preventive health care programs for the elderly have been nonexistent in the United States; health care has been geared toward cure rather than prevention and maintenance.

The growth of the 65 to 85 and older segment, chronic health problems, and government entitlement programs providing health insurance pose a tremendous problem for government funding. Quality issues are of great concern not only from an ethical standpoint with regard to care and treatment of the elderly but also from a cost vantage point.

❖ LEGISLATION AND ORGANIZATIONS TO AID THE ELDERLY

In the early part of the twentieth century the health needs of specific segments began to be recognized (see box on p. 198). The National Health Institute was established in 1930, and the first Social Security Amendment was enacted in 1935. Provisions of the Social Security Act made funding available to meet the needs of the elderly. Those provisions included retirement, benefits to survivors, widows, widowers, and dependent children, and disability benefits. Many boarding homes, a precursor to present-day nursing homes, were opened after the Social Security Amendment provided a funding source. Most of the first homes were opened by widowed or retired nurses.

The first meeting of the International Association of Gerontology occurred in 1950 in Belgium. In 1959 a Senate subcommittee reported findings of a study that indicated inconsistent interpretation of regulations governing nursing homes and inadequate care; much of the care was being provided by nonprofessionals.

The plight of the elderly was given attention between 1961-1971 by a series of White House Conferences on Aging. The American Association of Retired Persons (AARP) sponsored National Issue Forums to focus on the need to develop medical and social alternatives for the aged.

The Older Americans Act was passed in 1965, granting provisions for community service, employment research, and nutrition programs for the elderly. Another provision of the Act included a Bill of Rights.

Legislation/Organizations to Aid Elderly	
1930	National Health Institute
1935	Social Security Amendment
1950	International Association of Gerontology meets
1959	Senate subcommittee report on nursing home inconsistencies
1961-1971	White House Conference on Aging
1965	Older Americans Act
1966	Medicare/Medicaid enacted
1967	JCAHO introduces accreditation process for long-term care
1980	HCFA publishes proposed regulations to consolidate care planning into a single condition of participation
1987	Omnibus Budget Reconciliation Act (OBRA) passed. Mandates national use of minimum data set (MDS) for all patients whose reimbursement is from Medicare or Medicaid
1990	OBRA provisions implemented

In 1966 Medicare and Medicaid were enacted in an attempt to address the needs of the elderly. This enactment provided health insurance coverage for hospital, nursing home, skilled and unskilled care, and home health care. Medicare was oriented to acute or hospital and skilled nursing home or rehabilitative care. Medicare is financed by Social Security payments and administered by HCFA through the Department of Health and Human Services, formerly the Department of Health, Education, and Welfare (HEW). Medicare consists of Part A for acute care and Part B, a voluntary program funded by the enrollee paying one half and the government paying one half. Medicaid funding is administered by individual states and provides coverage for the indigent. Both Medicare and Medicaid payments are made by private companies under contract with government.

In 1967 the Joint Commission introduced its accreditation process for long-term care facilities, and the Comprehensive Older Americans Act was passed in 1978. Points of the Act included support for statewide long-term care advocacy programs, a provision for the introduction of senior centers, and the development of an Administration on Aging (AOA) in each state.

In 1980 HCFA published proposed regulations that would consolidate all resident care planning into a simple condition of participation, requiring patient assessments to be performed by a multidisciplinary team of health care providers. HCFA also contracted with the Institute on Medicine (IOM) to conduct studies of regulations governing nursing homes and make recommendations.

The Omnibus Budget Reconciliation Act was passed in 1987 and implemented in October 1990. This legislation established standards for nurses aide training, quality assessment activities, resident rights, and quality of life. OBRA also required Medicare certified nursing facilities to have a quality assurance committee composed of a director of nursing, administrator, physician, and three other staff members. OBRA 1987 mandated nursing homes have an RN on duty during the day for at least 8 hours, 7 days per week, and the development of comprehensive care plans.

In 1988 HCFA contracted with the Research Training Institute, the Hebrew Rehabilitation Center for the Aged, Brown University and the University of Michigan to develop a comprehensive resident assessment tool called the minimum data set (MDS).

OBRA law was geared toward improving quality of care and quality of life for nursing home residents. Under OBRA, patients' rights are to be promoted and protected, including the right to a dignified existence, self-determination, and communication with persons and services inside and outside the facility. Nursing homes are required to encourage participation in care planning, management of financial affairs, and choosing and contacting a MD. Facilities are required to develop policies and procedures for prevention of staff mistreatment. Care must promote maintenance or the enhancement of each patient's quality of life, and the environment must be safe, clean, and comfortable.

Under OBRA the resident assessment MDS must be performed on admission, at intervals throughout patient stay, and in the event of a significant change in condition. MDS emphasis is on a resident's capabilities before disabilities and the prevention of deterioration. Information for MDS is made through observation of the patient and interaction with family, significant others, and health care professionals and hospitals.

The MDS has four major goals. One is to develop an assessment that is standardized and fosters a new approach to the manner in which the information is analyzed. The use of the information is designed to improve the quality of life by improving the care planning process. Specific portions of the MDS must be completed on a quarterly basis, and a complete MDS must be done on every resident at least once a year. All minimum data sets must be easily retrieved up to 2 years after completion.

OBRA requires that the MDS be coordinated by a registered nurse and must include input from all appropriate health care personnel. The registered nurse is required to sign and certify the assessment and is subject to legal action if found falsifying information.

There are 18 resident assessment protocols (RAPs). The purpose of the RAP is to organize the data of the MDS and to assist the long-term care staff in thinking about the assessment and the care plan for each resident. RAP key instructions include clinical data and suggestions or approaches to care or additional assessment. Completion of the RAPs will key the long-term care staff into any unique problems or potential problems that may adversely affect the patient's highest level of functioning.

❖ OBRA AND DRUG UTILIZATION

Another major focus of the OBRA regulation is the use of drugs and, more specifically, psychotropic drugs. Drug reactions occur most often in long-term care facilities to residents who have multiple disease entities and medications. Statistical reports indicate that 75% of all drug interactions in long-term care could be avoided by adjustment of the dose, administration times, or the use of another drug. Most of the drug reactions occur with the old chronic care drugs such as digoxin, hypoglycemics, and warfarin. Those residents taking the greatest number of drugs are at the highest risk. When many drugs are prescribed for multiple therapeutic purposes, cumulative side effects may occur. Some of the more serious drug interactions with residents with multiple pathologies are the following:

1. Confusion, with loss of drug effectiveness
2. Confusion, with worsening of the disease
3. Drug-induced cardiovascular disease, myocardial ischemia
4. Electrolyte imbalance, altered thyroid functioning, and pulmonary disease
5. Alteration of food metabolism, and in turn, altering drug action
6. Interaction with diagnostic testing, therefore making interpretations more difficult

The OBRA law related to drug usage was a response to an Institute of Medicine report in 1986. OBRA states that the resident has the right to be free from any physical restraints or use of any psychoactive drug for the convenience of the staff, which is not required for treatment of medical symptoms. Unnecessary drug use is defined as those drugs given in excessive doses for excessive periods of time without a documented reason. They are considered unnecessary when an undue adverse consequence indicates that the dose should be reduced or the medication discontinued. Other unnecessary drugs are those prescribed in anticipation of a drug reaction.

Facilities are encouraged to work with physicians to prepare plans for gradual dosage reductions and behavioral programming to resolve suboptimal use of psychoactive medications. Gradual dosage reduction involves tapering the daily dosage, evaluating the resident's response to the tapering, determining if the resident can be managed on a lower dosage, or totally discontinuing the drug. Behavioral programming involves the modification of the resident's behavior, the environment, or both, to reduce behavioral disturbances. Discontinuance of an antipsychotic agent is contraindicated in a resident who has a documented need for the drug. The minimum dosage necessary to control the symptoms must be used.

There are many reasons for psychotropic drug misuse among the elderly. Often the elderly lack understanding of drug toxicities, staff inadequately differentiates between the origin of the problems and the symptoms of behavior disturbance, and the need exists for environmental control in a long-term care facility.

❖ TYPES OF INSTITUTIONAL CARE

There are various types of long-term care funded by differing services. Public care is sponsored by city, county, or state government and is financed through tax dollars. Historically, cost for care in public institutions is less.

Private nonprofit facilities are owned and operated by corporations, associations, religious, or other nonprofit groups. Funds for operation come through donations, grants, and patient fees. Profits do not benefit any one individual. The cost is usually higher than in public institutions.

Private for-profit facilities are owned and operated by individuals, partnerships, or corporations. Earnings are shared between owners, and the bulk of cost of care is paid by patient and family.

Facilities are licensed by individual states. State governments develop standards of care, survey institutions, and license the facility if it meets requirements. The state monitors compliance with periodic inspections.

Certified facilities are those that, in addition to licensure, desire certification. Facilities wanting to provide care to Medicare and Medicaid patients must meet additional standards and pass a state reviewing agency inspection.

Medicare skilled units are long-term care units in which patients need skilled services. Benefits are paid under Part A, and coverage is based on the need for daily skilled services such as skilled nursing or physical therapy.

Some facilities are dually certified to provide skilled services and what was formerly called *intermediate level care*. Since OBRA 1990 the distinction in dually certified facilities has been removed. Now patients are considered Level I or Level II, with Level I for those needing the least intensive care.

❖ QUALITY ASSESSMENT IN LONG-TERM CARE

Quality of care in nursing home settings is being examined by governmental agencies, third-party payors, and the news media. Various studies over the years have indicated the elderly's concern with quality of care and life. Nursing homes are a major provider of long-term care and are continually growing. Traditional nursing home care has been provided by nonprofessionals who lack quality pay and receive few benefits. Government has attempted to deal with staffing by requiring use of professional staff.

Elements of quality differ among groups, depending on who is the consumer. For patients, quality is often defined as staff responsiveness to their needs, courtesy of staff, relief of symptoms, and functional improvement. The purchaser of care such as an insurance company or third-party payor looks at efficiency and cost savings.

In long-term care, quality assessment must address quality of care and quality of life. *Quality of life* refers to the environment in which care is provided and is a multidimensional concept that looks at physical functioning, comfort, freedom of choice, and the emotional and social well-being of the resident.

The governing body is responsible for requiring and supporting an effective facility-wide quality assessment process. Administrative staff members are responsible for establishing and operating overall quality assessment processes, and individual departments are responsible for their components. The quality assessment process must include a written, comprehensive plan that describes its objectives, organization, and scope of practice with lines of communication and authority.

JCAHO introduced an accreditation program for long-term care in 1967. Since 1986 QA standards in long-term care have specified systematic monitoring and evaluation, important aspects of care that require a facility-wide, ongoing program.

JCAHO specifies nine components essential to quality assessment monitoring and evaluation in long-term care:
1. Responsibility
2. Scope of services
3. Aspects of care
4. Indicators
5. Measurements
6. Data collection
7. Corrective action
8. Evaluation of corrective action
9. Integration of information

Departments in which quality assessment should be developed in long-term care are medical records, nursing, activities, dietary, social services, maintenance, and administration.

Minutes of meetings must be kept, with introduction of problems, action, and follow-up.

❖ CQI - RESIDENT ASSESSMENT INSTRUMENT IN LONG-TERM CARE

Quality assessment has been established as an important part of health care. To go beyond traditional quality assessment, the incorporation of CQI in nursing homes is also a positive approach to enhancing quality. CQI requires ongoing inhouse measurement and, ideally, a national data base for comparative purposes. The resident assessment instrument, which is part of OBRA 1990, is being used nationally to assess nursing home residents and is an excellent source of data collection.

Defining quality in a nursing facility is difficult because of the varied ages of the residents. Some residents will stay only a few months, whereas others will spend a year or more. Severely demented residents often coexist with residents with physical impairment only. All of this makes it difficult for the organization to clearly delineate its mission and service goals, which is an essential step in quality care.

Donabedian's model of three approaches to quality, structure, process, and outcome traditionally applied to primary medical care can be applied to long-term care units. The use of structure, process, and outcome can combine a large number of variables and can be combined in an infinite variety. Structure represents the institution's capacity to provide care; process defines services and resource utilization; and outcomes reflect consequence, although applied to long-term care, comparative analysis is difficult.

In 1989 Glass defined quality nursing home care as:

> ... the degree to which appropriate services are provided in a safe and clean environment, whereby residents achieve and maintain maximal levels of functional independence, and best possible control of physical/organic health conditions, and whereby the importance of the individual is recognized, and positive feelings, self-confidence, and the dignity of residents is supported.

The ability of nursing homes to clearly understand their organization and how it functions has been severely lacking. In addition, the nursing home is a specialized setting in which quality of care and quality of life are uniquely and tightly intertwined.

Studies of residents, their families, and data from researchers indicate that quality must go beyond the traditional medical model and include an environment supportive of autonomy, psychosocial aspects such as staff attitudes, and ties with the community.

A broader vision of quality is addressed by Glass in a conceptual model. This model includes four major dimensions of nursing home quality: staff intervention, physical environment, food/nutrition, and community relations. The RAI is an excellent source of data to measure these indicators of quality.

Through the use of the resident assessment instrument and additional refinements, national data can be collected and norms established for national use. Norms could eventually be replaced by standards set by expert opinion. Adding indicators for care to the present system would provide additional information to standardize data.

Process and outcome variables linked to nursing home quality can be readily retrieved from the RAI, which paves the way to a new era of increased knowledge regarding nursing homes. Before instituting the RAI little tangible data were available. This lack of data has severely impaired nursing home staff in trying to pursue CQI activities. Industry performance based standards are critical in pursuance of CQI in the long-term care setting and can pave the way toward emphasis on positive incentives for providers offering good care. These homes would be regarded with less expensive and less frequent surveys and more leverage with experimentation with innovative approaches.

❖ UTILIZATION MANAGEMENT IN LONG-TERM CARE

Resource utilization is as important in the long-term care setting as in any other. Increasing use of long-term care units and greater government expenditures for long-term care make control of resources essential for long-term viability of facilities. The goal of utilization management in long-term care should be to maintain high quality patient care and effective use of resources. The utilization plan is subject to approval of a licensing or a certifying agency. A utilization committee should review extended stays, discharge plans, and medical evaluations. The UM committee should review the UM plan and make recommendations to the governing body and administration.

❖ INFECTION CONTROL IN LONG-TERM CARE

The JCAHO requires each long-term care facility to have a facility-wide program for surveillance, prevention, and control of infection. All patient care or support departments are required to participate.

There should be written policies and procedures covering the role and scope of each department's participation in prevention and control activities and types of surveillance used to monitor rates of nosocomial infections. Activities must be conducted to prevent and control infections in patients and personnel. Supervision of the program includes representatives from at least the medical staff, nursing, administration, and persons responsible for the infection control program.

With the inception of DRGs many people are leaving the acute care setting in need of lower levels of care. The long-term care unit serves as this level of care for many. Sicker patients mean patients requiring more care, with a greater risk for infections. A well-defined and well-implemented infection control program will be critical for long-term care facilities. In facilities where rooms are semiprivate or in ward settings, infection control practices that prevent the spread of infection are critical. Staff education will be very important in control of infection. Infections in long-term care units can become epidemic to staff and other patients. Infections can prolong nursing home stays, hamper recovery, and increase resource utilization and readmissions to acute care.

❖ RISK MANAGEMENT IN LONG-TERM CARE

The shifting of sicker patients to long-term care, governmental, media, and public scrutiny of elderly care, and growing numbers of aged will affect risk management in long-term care facilities. Establishment of national standards of care provide a basis for risk management issues and the potential for lawsuits when guidelines are not followed. The restrictions on psychotropic drug use and restraints, although in one sense helpful and appropriate for patients, create the potential for adverse occurrences and subsequent lawsuits. Diversification of services and use of technology in long-term care also creates the potential for adverse occurrences. Continued shifting of care to alternate delivery systems such as long-term care will by sheer numbers create risk exposures. Occurrence reporting will be beneficial and necessary for quality assessment monitoring and evaluation activities.

Staffing in nursing homes will become a greater issue as the needs of a wide variety of persons are identified. Nonprofessional staff historically have cared for nursing home patients. Lower pay and few benefits, commonplace traditionally in nursing homes, will hamper the ability to attract qualified professional staff. These issues will pose a serious risk.

❖ IMPLICATIONS FOR NURSING PRACTICE

Greater numbers of nurses will be needed to care for the growing numbers of elderly in nursing homes. Quality of care will continue to be a concern, and nursing will be the hub from which all care planning will originate. Facilities will be challenged to provide competitive salaries and benefit packages to attract qualified nursing professionals. Nursing and technical skills will continue to be important as acuity of patients increases and greater technology is offered in the nursing home setting.

OBRA places the registered nurse in the role of coordinator of the resident assessment instrument. The responsibility for completion of accurate data is placed on the registered nurse. The use of the MDS aids the nurse in nursing process, assessing, planning, implementing, and re-evaluating. Nursing will continue to use skills of nursing judgment in working with all patients but especially those who have multifaceted disease processes and reside in the home over a long period. Nursing staff members, in their role as coordinator of care, will be uniquely positioned to determine when patients are nearing discharge potential or require another level of care. Nursing is key to quality of care and quality of life concerns in long-term care settings and can play a leading role working with quality management and into continuous quality improvement.

❖ FUTURE OF LONG-TERM CARE

Since the inception of DRGs and prospective payment for acute care, patients have shifted from the acute care setting to alternate levels of care. Long-term care has served as an alternative delivery setting. Often patients leave acute care, requiring continued rehabilitation or follow-up but are not ill enough to remain in the acute care setting. Long-term care serves as a level of care appropriate for these types of patients, and many are using the services. This trend is expected to continue as the numbers of elderly grow. Long-term care units will also be used for those patients who have chronic illness, requiring ongoing medical treatment and nursing intervention. Case management companies charged with the responsibility of lowering costs while guiding the patient through a course of illness will be especially interested in what long-term care units have to offer.

Long-term care will continue to become more complex as the consumers of the care become more varied in needs. An integrated, well-organized quality management team will become critical as the complexity increases. Integrated quality management can also serve as the trainers and initiators of quality as the facility, as a whole, begins the CQI process. Because government expenditures support much of the long-term care industry, continuous quality improvement will be of even greater importance as facilities strive to give high quality care and reduce cost.

❖ SUMMARY

The numbers of persons 65 years of age or older requiring health care are increasing. As longevity increases, the elderly are concerned with the quality of their lives. Long-term care units serve as one level of care not only for those needing short-term skilled services after an acute illness but also for those needing care from months to years. OBRA 1987 dealt with many issues related to quality of life and quality of care and, most notably, required all facilities who accept Medicare and Medicaid patients to use a resident assessment tool nationally in assessing and reassessing patients. This was the first comprehensive, standardized assessment tool for long-term care facilities. OBRA also removed the distinction between skilled units and intermediate level units. Now patients are Level I or Level II. Quality management and continuous quality improvement will become increasingly more important as greater numbers of persons with varied needs are placed in the long-term care setting. Nursing is the center from which all care planning originates and can be a catalyst in the overall CQI movement. The minimum data set or resident assessment instrument will be the beginning for the accumulation of data on a national scale for quality of care and life issues and can help identify processes through which CQI can be improved.

REFERENCES

1. American Society of Consultant Pharmacists, *Guidelines for use of behavior modifying drugs in long-term care facilities*, 3, 1988.
2. Birchinall JM, Straight ME: *The care of the older adult*, Philadelphia, 1982, JB Lippincott.
3. Burnside IM: *Nursing and the aged*, New York, 1982, McGraw-Hill.
4. Clark MJD: *Health care for today and tomorrow*, Reston, Va, 1984, Reston Publishing.
5. Futrell M et al: *Primary health care of the older adult*, Boston, 1980, Duxbury Press.
6. Greatting-Haydon S: Meeting the new long-term care facility participation requirements for medication restraints, *Consultant Pharmacist*, 680, December 1989.
7. Griffin K: Changes in resident profile present many opportunities, *Provider*, 9, July 1990.
8. McLeod K: AHCA largest providers: "make best use of OBRA," *Provider*, 9, July 1990.
9. Morris JN et al: Designing the national resident assessment instrument for nursing homes, *Gerentologist* 30(3):293, 1990.
10. Sherman R: New regulations require preparation, *Contemporary Long-Term Care*, p 79, February 1990.

CHAPTER
15

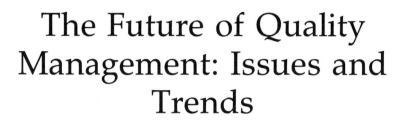

The Future of Quality Management: Issues and Trends

THE issues and trends of quality management in health care are numerous. Today's consumers and health care providers are more educated and more concerned about "quality" in their health care services. This chapter will highlight a few of the many current trends that nursing professionals will encounter in today's practice environment while they improve patient care through integrated quality management.

❖ RESEARCH

Research is becoming more important to basic practice in clinical nursing. Although nursing administrators must support research, not all nurses will actually perform it. However, every nurse must have the knowledge to interpret research and apply it to practice. Nurses, in this way, are both consumers and producers of research. Research must be the cornerstone for decision making in the work place.

Quality management interfaces well with professional nursing research. Quality assessment and improvement committees can use research as a primary approach to achieving positive patient outcomes. Data collection and analysis are important to research, as well as integrated quality management. Monitoring and evaluating *infection control* data, *utilization management* issues, *risk* and *safety* information, and *quality assessment* studies all have some implications for research. In today's environment quality management can identify nursing practice problems that are best addressed through research.

Research can help nurses document both social and clinical efficiency of professional practice to third-party payors, consumers, and regulatory groups such as the federal government. Research can help assess the effectiveness of nursing actions in patient care. Nursing research can demonstrate that nurses can make a difference and produce positive patient care outcomes. Research can be used to improve the use of resources and decrease costs[7] (Fig. 15-1). Nurses can improve the quality of patient care through integrated quality management approaches that are research based.

The research presently done by nurses in areas of health promotion is important. As nurses document the affect of exercise, healthful nutritional patterns, nonsmoking, and breast self-examination on preventing illness, insurance companies will see that their dollars are better spent on prevention rather than treatment (*utilization management*). Prevention of infection, such as teaching safer sex and universal precautions, can perhaps affect the continuing devastation that AIDS has had in this country (*infection control*). This will decrease costs of treatment through prevention (*utilization management*). Research on high-risk populations may change the course of illness (*risk management*) and produce positive health care outcomes (*quality assessment and improvement*). In so many ways quality management has a direct relationship to nursing research.

Research can be related to ethics, another area of nursing practice in which integrated quality management is essential. The concept of *beneficence*, or the risk-benefit ratio, is an important part of medical ethics. The researcher must be prepared to discontinue the research if there is undue harm or distress put on the subjects. The general guideline is that the risk should never exceed the expected humanitarian benefits or knowledge desired. Other ethical issues related to research include informed consent, confidentiality and anonymity, and fair treatment.[13]

Several models have been proposed for effective use of nursing research in quality improvement. Fig. 15-2[7] and 15-3[14] demonstrate two approaches to this process. The nurse administrator who supports quality care will also view research as essential to professional practice, which involves staff at all levels in improving practice. Research-based practice provided through the integrated quality management process will secure respect for the contribu-

> **Clinical problem:** The nurse works on a surgical unit where many heparin locks are used as an intermittent infusion device. The hospital routine is to use heparin 10 units every 8 hours and after each medication administration to flush the lock. The nurse reads a research study that identifies that saline flush is as effective as heparin flush in maintaining patency and preventing phlebitis in peripheral heparin locks.
>
> | Individual process | Organizational process |
> |---|---|
> | Reads research article | Reads research article |
> | Discusses article with peers on unit | Discusses article with research utilization committee |
> | Approaches nurse manager about changing procedure for flushing peripheral heparin locks | Committee proceeds with research utilization and asks staff nurse to participate |
> | Believes a standardized approach should be used for all patients having heparin locks and is unsure if children should be included | Research utilization activities involve (1) gathering studies related to heparin lock flush, (2) critiquing them, (3) establishing a research base, (4) translating findings into a new research-based procedure for flushing heparin locks, (5) providing inservices for nursing, pharmacy, and physicians to explain new procedure and reason for practice change, (6) implementing the new saline flush procedure for adult patients, and (7) evaluating the outcome |
> | Assumes responsibility and accountability for implementation and for evaluating patient outcomes | |
>
> Outcomes of using this new procedure were:
>
> 1. Elimination of risks to heparin. Heparin-induced thrombocytopenia, thrombus, hemorrhage, and medication incompatibilities were eliminated, thereby improving the quality of patient care.
>
> 2. A significant cost savings by eliminating heparin as the flush solution. A savings in nursing time occurred because of the elimination of the need to flush before and after administration of drugs incompatible with heparin. In addition, an annual savings of $38,000 was realized by using saline instead of heparin.
>
> This is only one example of a significant contribution that research has made to health care.

FIGURE 15-1
Comparison of individual and organizational approach to research utilization. (From Goode C, Bulechek GM: Research utilization: an organizational process that enhances quality of care, *J Nurs Care Qual*, Special Report, 1992, p. 34.)

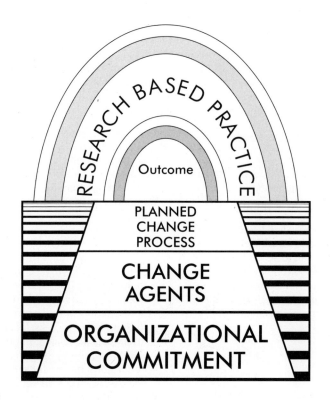

FIGURE 15-2
An organizational process research utilization model. (From Goode C, Bulechek GM: Research Utilization: an organizational process that enhances quality of care, *J Nurs Care Qual*, Special Report, 1992, p. 27.)

tion nursing makes in managing resources, infections, risks, safety, and improving quality.

Nursing administrators must foster the climate that encourages creativeness for research, stimulating intellectual pursuits of research and dedicating the resources needed to perform this work. The integrated processes of quality management must be included in the research performed in the practice setting. There must also be rewards for utilization of research in all settings of nursing practice.

Research utilization must be seen as necessary to quality in nursing practice. Through integrated quality management processes, research can monitor and evaluate patient care outcomes. Studies must include cost effectiveness of nursing practices, as well as the implications for risk and

CHAPTER 15 THE FUTURE OF QUALITY MANAGEMENT: ISSUES AND TRENDS

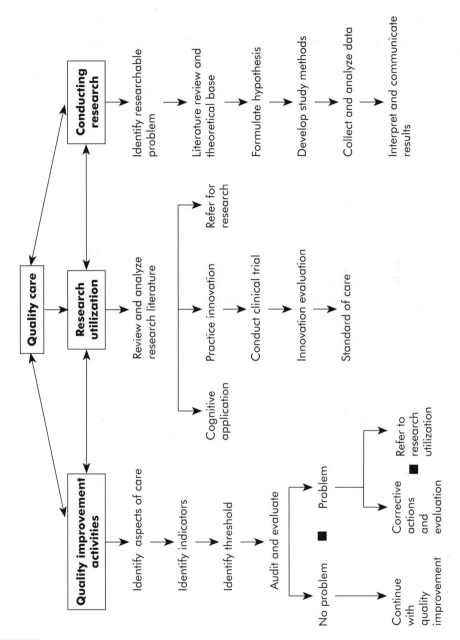

FIGURE 15-3
Charleston area medical center research-based nursing practice model. (From Rosswurm MA: A research-based practice model in a hospital setting, *J Nurs Adm* 22(3):59, 1992.)

patient safety. Agencies that encourage research and evaluation in all areas of *quality management*—infection control, risk and safety, utilization management, and quality assessment—will have the competitive edge in both recruitment and retention of professional staff and in preferred provider relationships with third-party payors.

❖ ETHICS

Bioethics is the term used to describe the application of ethics to human life in society. The term means *life ethics* and is usually interchanged with the term *medical ethics*. It is a large area of concern in today's health care environment that includes topics related to the following[16]:

1. Mercy killing, mercy death, euthanasia
2. Treatment of dying patients
3. Birth control, sterilization, and abortion
4. Human experimentation and informed consent
5. Genetics, fertilization, and birth
6. Organ transplantation
7. Confidentiality in professional relationships
8. Allocation of scarce health care resources

The "Right to Die"

All states have laws recognizing the right of the patient to make health care decisions, including refusal of medical care. However, the Cruzan case has brought more interest about this constitutional right. On June 25, 1990, the U.S. Supreme Court issued the first "right-to-die" decision in the case of Nancy Cruzan. Basically the Court upheld the right of a competent person to refuse life-sustaining treatment such as nutrition or hydration. It also held that the states could determine the degree of proof necessary before the patient's wishes would be followed. This "proof" would be in the form of an advance directive.

The Patient Self Determination Act is most important because it defines the legal obligations of health care agencies concerning the right to die. The Act imposes new regulations on health care providers that receive federal funding through Medicare and Medicaid to protect the patient's rights. The Act also encourages patients to review and document treatment options before becoming incapacitated. Although the patient may waive the right to an advanced directive, evidence that the patient was given adequate information to make an informed decision must be in the medical record. This increases the patient's opportunity to receive and understand this information. Written information must be given to all adult patients on admission or on receipt of care in all settings from hospital to home care. The basic message from Congress is clear: Patients must be informed of their rights, and federally funded health care providers must provide patients with their rights.[9]

The right-to-die issue has drawn attention to Washington state. In 1991 voters almost approved legislation allowing doctors to legally administer lethal injections or use other means to assist a terminally ill patient to die. This could be the first site in the world to legalize physician-assisted suicide, although the Netherlands unofficially permits it. Opponents disagree with the moral and ethical implications of this legislation. Some consider it contrary to the principle of respect for human life. Basically this initiative would allow physicians to assist the terminal patient in death if the patient is mentally competent. The patient must have been diagnosed by two doctors and have a prognosis of 6 months or less. The request must be in writing and witnessed by two disinterested parties. The physician, nurses, hospital, and/or nursing homes would be immune from liability whether or not they comply with the patient's wishes.[12]

Although the American Medical Association (AMA) has no formal position on this subject, some physicians think it violates the AMA Code of Ethics. They suggest a better solution is good pain management. The impact of such proposed initiatives, whether enacted or not, point to the increasing emphasis on bioethics in today's world.

"The Gag Rule"

The Supreme Court decision in the Rust *v.* Sullivan case places professional nurses in violation with the American Nurses Association (ANA) Code of Ethics. The Supreme Court has ruled that clinics receiving funds under Title X cannot discuss abortion with patients, even if requested. This forces nurses to give different kinds of care, especially in the area of informed consent.

The decision has been challenged in five areas:
1. Congressional intent in creating the program (Title X)
2. Free speech on the part of the health care professional

3. Separation of facilities
4. Doctor-patient relationship/doctor's silence acting as a barrier to health care
5. Fifth Amendment right to privacy and abortion

The ANA Statement on Reproductive Health states the patient has a right to privacy and the right to make informed decisions based on full information, without coercion. It also reinforces the obligation of health care professionals to share any relevant information about the client's legal choices. The statement further explains that if the state limits this right to information and informed decision, an unethical restraint will jeopardize the provider-client relationship.

The AMA concurs with the ANA, condemning any government interference with the physician-patient relationship in which the physician's judgment is compromised by withholding information. The National League for Nursing (NLN) shares this viewpoint, stating that deliberate withholding of information would be contrary to the best interest of the patient and would refute the patient's right to informed decision making.

All three professional groups believe this will precipitate a two-tiered health care system. Those who can pay will have access to information, whereas those using federally funded clinics will be denied this information. The ethical issue is whether the government has the right to censor information about choices to the patients receiving federally funded health care. The ultimate concern is whether freedom of speech is a fundamental right in the United States.[6]

Mandatory Testing and Disclosure of HIV

The ANA has issued a statement reaffirming the commitment of the organization to quality patient care. The ANA does not support mandatory testing and disclosure of HIV status because this will not prevent the spread of HIV. Only strict adherence to universal precautions and infection control measures will curtail HIV transmission.

ANA opposes mandatory testing on several grounds. Testing is not always reliable and is expensive. A negative test today may not be the same in a month. There is simply no way to monitor HIV except through personal responsibility. Spread of HIV can be stopped through consumer education and safe infection control practices.

ANA supports the patient's right to protection from AIDS. This can be accomplished by broad dissemination of information outlining strict infection control principles that must be used by health care workers. Federally set guidelines should be monitored and enforced. Nationally set standards should be set for invasive procedures. All health care settings including outpatient and physician offices should be subject to inspection.

This statement supports the ANA Code of Ethics that expects the nurse to safeguard the client and the public when health care and safety are affected because nurses are patient advocates and their safety and well-being are the primary concern in nursing care delivery. Confidentiality must be considered. Voluntary testing and disclosure of the nurse's status is encouraged, as well as reporting the patient's status when a nurse has been exposed to a HIV patient's body fluids.[18]

Implications for Quality Management

All components of integrated quality management are significant. Each situation has elements of *risk* and *safety* both to the consumer and to the professional nurse. Ethical decisions will indeed affect the use and allocation of resources, which is a form of *utilization management*. Organ transplants and HIV transmission issues will rely on *infection control* principles and enforcement. Positive or adverse outcomes will be documented through monitoring and evaluation in *quality assessment* studies. Ethics is certainly an area in which integrated quality management in nursing practice in any setting can make a difference.

❖ THIRD-PARTY REVIEW AND PAYORS

As more emphasis is placed on appropriate health care services at cost-efficient rates, third-party payors will affect the health care delivery system. When defining the *external customers* nurses must address to provide quality care, these parties are among the most influential. In a time when dollars spent on health care are controlled by demonstration of positive patient care outcomes, the professional nurse has a great opportunity to show worth.

This is especially true for advanced practice nurses such as nurse practitioners. Although legislation is present for direct reimbursement to nurses, implementing this is more difficult. As the third-party payors look for more efficient ways to spend their limited health care dollars, securing direct reimbursement can be a reality.

One way to demonstrate the cost efficiency of nursing care is with research based on quality management processes. Can the nurse show effective use of limited resources with positive patient outcomes through *utilization management* and *quality assessment?* Are nurse practitioners documenting their impact on health promotion and *infection control problems?* Are studies available to describe how nurses affect the *safety* and minimize *risks* to patients? In short how have nurses demonstrated they can make a difference in quality patient care delivery? Integrated quality management practices will enhance the probability and increase opportunities to receive health care reimbursement.

❖ HIGH TECHNOLOGY

One fact is inevitable for nursing: technology continues to improve choices for health care services delivery. This impacts the nurse in many ways. The use of technology has many implications for integrated quality management.

High-Technology Home Care

High technology has been accepted as part of acute care for some time. In fact many patients went to the hospital because they needed the high technology that only the acute care setting could provide. Today many of the same services once considered safe only in acute care are being delivered in the home. These include intravenous antibiotics, total parenteral nutrition (TPN), intravenous dobutamine, chemotherapy, and intravenous blood products.

Home care is usually less costly than the acute care setting. The patient and family assume responsibility for care, and the cost of continuous nursing is eliminated. The family must learn to administer the therapy and change dressings in an acceptable way, using sterile technique. The home care nurse is usually available at the start of service on an intermittent basis and then checks on the patient's progress throughout therapy, drawing laboratory work.

The nurse must integrate quality management principles into the plan of care. By using home care, health care resources are better spent, which is a part of *utilization management.* The nurse must teach patient and family *infection control* principles, as well as monitor for any signs and symptoms of infection. There are many *risks* in delivering high technology in an uncontrolled setting such as the home, but the nurse teaches *safety* to the patient and family to minimize these. *Quality assessment* is necessary to monitor and evaluate clinical patient outcomes and maintain the patient safely in the home environment.

The nurse administrator uses quality management in deciding if the particular staff member has the competency to provide the high-tech intravenous care. Resources must be provided and dollars budgeted for the education nursing staff needs to meet the growing high-tech needs in home care. The nurse administrator must assess each case for quality issues, without pressures from insurers, physicians, and senior administration.

Computerization

Computerization can assist the nurse administrator in controlling and planning management functions. As nurses know, collecting data and analyzing information are major and critical parts of planning. The nurse must work to transform data into a meaningful form to manage daily operations, whatever the setting.

A frequent problem with computerization in nursing is the intimidation the nurse may experience. Perhaps the nurse does not have the ability to type and feels threatened by the keyboard often used with computers. Some nurses fear loss of their job if unable to adapt to computerization. The nurse administrator must help staff members overcome this fear by being a role model in effective use of computerization.

What are the benefits of computerization? One major benefit is the establishment of a comprehensive data base used to accomplish the following:
1. Monitor patient acuity and adjust staffing
2. Plan and maintain a budget
3. Record and update inservice education programs for staff
4. Provide individualized learning programs for staff
5. Provide consistent quality patient education tools
6. Assist with discharge planning
7. Provide information for planning patient care

Computer programs may stimulate new thoughts and approaches. They provide immediate reward with a printout of the screen, if desired. In an environment with restricted resources, computers can help nursing administrators and staff use resources wisely.[18]

At Walter Reed Army Medical Center computers have improved patient care outcomes through patient education. A study was conducted that included 52 asthmatic patients ages 18 to 75. The majority had some experience in using a computer. A computer program, called Avoidance Measures in House Dust Mite Allergy, was used by these patients rather than use of traditional education, written materials, and counseling.

The patient care outcomes assessed were the following: (1) adherence to implementing avoidance measures; (2) home dust mite allergen levels in mattresses, bedroom, and living room carpets; and (3) symptomatology. The computer group had a significantly higher adherence level after using the computer program for self-education. The computer group also had a significantly lower level of home dust mite allergens. Again the computer educated group had lower symptomatology and a greater reduction in the use of inhaled bronchodilators.[10]

These results demonstrate that positive patient outcomes may be achieved with the assistance of computerized programs in patient education. The quality of the patient's care was improved through use of advanced technology.

Computers are most useful to integrated quality management. *Risk* and *safety* data can be collected and trended. *Quality assessment* data can be aggregated for analysis and improvement of care. *Infection control* surveillance reports become more manageable with computerization. Labor intensive reports that were once prepared manually can be produced more often for better use in management and operations. A good example of *utilization management* is the ability to remove babies from sleep apnea monitors sooner because of a computerized detection monitor.[17] Data can be rapidly accessed to free the nurse for patient care. This allows better plans of care and improved patient care outcomes. Computerization used in a judicious way clearly is an outstanding way to advance nursing quality management activities and improve patient care.

❖ MARKETING

As the health care dollars dwindle, providers are competing for increased health care market share. Marketing is an important part of strategic planning, which is the role of the nurse administrator. The ultimate goal of marketing is to develop strategies that will help the organization meet its objectives.[8] Marketing must start by identifying the needs, preferences, and perceptions of the customers, both internal and external. Internal customers include the patient, physicians, other professionals, and organization departments. External customers include the community, visitors, suppliers, and payors.[2]

Integrating quality management into the marketing plan can help accomplish many management objectives. Quality management requires measuring outcomes, or defining "starting" and "desired" values. The nurse administrator can then measure progress of quality improvement efforts by analyzing use of services, revenues, and expenses, employee satisfaction and turnover rates, inservice education attendance, and patient compliance and satisfaction.

Product line management has become increasingly popular in the past decade. The product line strategy means coordinating specific nursing areas with allied health providers to provide a more focused service, targeting patients, physicians, or payors.[1] This may be a specific area of nursing practice, such as oncology or pulmonary services. A nurse can best manage this product line because he or she has the continuous contact with the customers and is most knowledgeable about the product. This uses the specialized skills of the nurse and consequently increases productivity, satisfaction, and quality. As product managers use integrated quality management to demonstrate positive patient care outcomes, the consumer is attracted to that agency. "Quality" attracts payors and rewards agencies with preferred provider arrangements.[4]

Marketing the results of quality improvement can build loyalty in both internal and external customers. Marketing "quality" may not only increase market share but also may help to recruit and maintain nursing staff. Marketing an improved service is an excellent way to create new customers and maintain previous ones. Marketing and quality improvement must become interrelated in the organization if it is to be successful.

The following benefits result from integrating quality management into the marketing plan[15]:

1. Improved image for nursing
2. Ability of profession to attract qualified candidates for nursing preparation and retention of existing staff
3. Secure respect of other health care professionals and administrators for nursing as vital to organizational survival
4. Conducting nurse-driven marketing research with appropriate dissemination of results

❖ SUPPLEMENTAL STAFFING AGENCIES

With fluctuations in census and seasonal changes in nursing manpower needs, the nurse administrator may resort to the use of supplemental staffing agencies to complete the staffing pattern needed to provide patient care. Fortunately many nurses want to work part-time or to choose their own schedule. This provides a pool of nurses for supplemental staffing in the various settings.

The JCAHO has expressed concern over the responsibility the agency retains in providing quality care. The patient must receive the same quality care that a staff member of the agency would be expected to give. The nurse administrator must carefully examine the reputation of the staffing agency and question the records maintained to document competent staff. The nurse administrator can request that the agency have staff trained in the quality management processes that employed staff maintain. Policies and procedures crucial to *infection control, risk* and *safety management, utilization management,* and *quality assessment* must be shared with agency staff, with defined expectations. Confidentiality concerns must be discussed. In short the conscientious nurse administrator must critique the agency staff to maintain the expected high level of integrated quality management.

❖ NURSING AGENDA FOR HEALTH CARE REFORM

More than 40 nursing organizations have joined the ANA in endorsing the *Nursing Agenda for Health Care Reform*. In the executive summary the ANA acknowledges that nurses in the United States have always supported access, quality, and health care services at affordable costs. In a time of skyrocketing costs and decreased access to quality care, nursing has defined an Agenda for immediate reform. Many of the core tenets interface well with integrated quality management.

The Agenda would provide a restructured health care system that would foster utilization of the "most cost-effective providers and therapeutic options in the most appropriate settings" (utilization management). A public plan would be devised to provide coverage for the poor, small businesses, and individuals at risk because of preexisting conditions such as AIDS (risk management and infection control). Steps to reduce costs include use of managed care and case management, prudent resource allocation, and development of health care policies based on effectiveness and outcomes research (quality assessment and utilization management).[3]

In synopsis the Agenda is supported by integrated quality management processes with the goal of cost-effective quality care through the following[3]:
1. Provider availability
2. Consumer involvement
3. Outcome and effectiveness measures
4. Review mechanisms
5. Managed care
6. Case management

The ANA states that the existing health care system is a patched program that needs restructuring and reform. The time has come for a new vision led by American nurses. This vision must include the entire Agenda and integrated quality management.

❖ FUTURE OF INTEGRATED QUALITY MANAGEMENT

The future of integrated quality management promises to address current and future trends in health care delivery. It is paramount that nursing embrace the future, armed with the skills necessary to not only provide but also *demonstrate* quality care. Quality management processes such as infection control, quality assessment, utilization management, and risk and safety management must be part of each nurse's knowledge base and practice.

The nurse administrator of the future must be a visionary who uses the tools of quality improvement to better nursing practice and patient care in all settings. The climate necessary for integrated quality management must be fostered with resources and moral support to the practicing nurse. The nurse administrator will define the future of the practice in any setting, and he or she must be the role model for supporting integrated quality management. When this is true, the consumer, which includes every American, can expect to receive cost-effective quality nursing services in the most appropriate setting, with demonstrated positive patient care outcomes.

REFERENCES

1. Alexander J, Robison BR: Positioning your nursing organization for product-line structure, *Nurs Admin Q* 15(2):49–52, 1991.
2. Alward RR: A marketing approach to nursing administration. I. *J Nurs Adm* 13(3):9–21, March 1983.
3. American Nurses Association: *Nursing's agenda for health care reform*, PR-3 220M, June 1991.

4. Bird GA: Product-line management and nursing, *Nursing Management* 19(5):46–48, May 1988.
5. Daughtery AN: Free speech denied, *The Tennessee Nurse* 54(4):25, Aug 1991.
6. Fagin CM: The economic value of nursing research, *Am J Nurs* 82(12):1844–1849, 1982.
7. Goode C, Bulechek GM: Research utilization: an organizational process that enhances quality of care, *J Nurs Care Qual*, special report:27–35, 1992, Aspen Publishers.
8. Hillstad SG, Berkowitz EN: Health care marketing plans: from strategy to action, 1991, Aspen Publishers.
9. Huntington SR, Fry-Revere S: Provider responsibilities under the patient self determination act—living wills, durable powers of attorney and the law. *Health Law Trends*, Winter 1991.
10. Huss K and others: Computer education for asthmatics: what effects? *J Nurs Care Qual* 6(3):57–66, 1992.
11. Joel L: *Statement by Lucille Joel on AIDS to the ANA house of delegates*, June 30, 1991.
12. Mayer D: Doc-aided suicide faces woes, *Healthweek* 5(12):5, June 17, 1991.
13. Polit DF, Hungler BP: *Essentials of nursing research*, ed 2, Philadelphia, JB Lippincott, 1989.
14. Rosswurm MA: A research-based practice model in a hospital setting, *J Nurs Adm* 22(3): 57–60, 1992.
15. Stanton M, Stanton G: Marketing nursing: model for success, *Nurs Management* 19(9): 36–38, 1988.
16. Thiroux JP: *Ethics: theory and practice,* ed 3, New York, 1986, MacMillian.
17. Thomas M: Computers free nurses for care, *The American Nurse,* p 1–2, July/Aug 1991.
18. Walters S: Computerized care plans help nurses achieve quality patient care, *J Nurs Adm* 16(11):33–39, Nov 1986.
19. Weiland DE: Can there be mutual support between hospital marketing and continuous quality improvement? *Journal for Healthcare Quality,* 14(1):30–31, 1992.

Glossary

admission review: performed within 24 hours of hospital admission; utilization function
advisory committee: group of agency, nonagency, and consumers that reviews policies/procedures and the overall operation of a HH agency
AHA: American Hospital Association
appropriateness evaluation protocol (AEP): appropriateness decision based on medical records information for surgery patients; utilization function
capitated payment: payment preset
Case Mix: combination of clinical and financial information, interpreted in numbers
CDC: Centers for Disease Control
certified: licensed and meets additional standards specified by federal regulations; passes an inspection to become certified
CHAMPUS: Civilian Health and Medical Programs for Uniformed Services insurance plan
comorbidity: complicating factor
certificate of need (CON): justification of need for capital expansion by a health care facility for need to build a facility or add a service
concurrent review: review for medical record for need and appropriateness of care; utilization function
deemed status: federal recognition of an organization's standards as being a benchmark of quality
diagnosis specific criteria: justify admission by reviewing patient's history, physical and emergency room record and, validating need for admission; utilization function
DRG: Diagnostic Related Group
DRG validation: determining if appropriate DRG assigned based on diagnosis
dually eligible: refers to patients who meet requirements to get both Medicare and Medicaid
economic stabilization program: attempt by Nixon 1972-1974 to control hospital rates
empirical: based on actual practice of professionals

epidemiology: the study of factors that contribute to the incidence, distribution, and control of disease, defect, disability, and death
fee for service: provider establishes a fee for service rendered
fiscal intermediary (FI): public or private groups designated by federal government to process health care claims and make payment for services
focused review: focus on specific issue; utilization function
Health Care Quality Improvement Act (HCQI): centralized data bank as a source of information regarding health care providers
Hill-Burton Act: federal funding for building hospitals
HMO: Health Maintenance Organization
home health nursing: a component of community health, incorporating both preventive and curative nursing
hospital-based home health agency: a division of a hospital
invasive procedure review: review of patients who had invasive procedures; utilization function
IPA: Individual Practice Association
length of stay (LOS): Age, single/multiple diagnosis or surgeries, and aggregate numbers of inpatient days based on regional data to establish norms for inpatient stays per DRG
licensed facility: licensed by the state based on standards set by state
loss exposure analysis: identify and estimate the likely significance of a potential loss
managed care: arrangement of comprehensive care that is coordinated, efficient, and cost effective
MDC: major diagnostic category
MDS: minimum data set; a basic assessment used in long-term care units
Medicare Part A: covers hospital, skilled nursing care, in a long-term care unit
Medicare Part B: voluntary; one half paid by federal funds and one half paid by patient; covers physician visits and some outpatient services
National Health Planning and Resources Development Act: established certificate of need (CON) requirements
normative criteria: based on professional opinion; relates to utilization
nosocomial: hospital-acquired infection
OBRA: Omnibus Budget Reconciliation Act
official health agencies: divisions of state and local health departments funded through state and local taxes
outlier review: review when patient is hospitalized more days than DRG specified or when cost is greater than preset amount; utilization function
pandemic: widespread epidemic of an infectious disease
patient classification system: means of classifying patient conditions
PPO: Preferred Provider Organization

PPS: Prospective Pricing—preset price
prepaid health programs: insurance companies where premiums are prepaid
principal diagnosis: condition largely responsible for admission to an acute care facility
principal procedure: procedure performed for treatment that is most closely related to principal diagnosis
private home health agencies or nursing homes: owned by individuals or corporations
private for-profit: agencies or facilities owned and operated by individual partnerships or corporations; earnings shared; bulk of cost paid by patient/family
private non-profit: agencies or facilities owned and operated by associations, religions, or other nonprofit groups; funded through donations, grants, and patient fees; profits do not benefit a single individual
PRO: Peer Review Organization
prospective review: review of proposed care; utilization function
public care: funded by taxpayers' dollars, sponsored by city, county, or state
provisional diagnosis: preliminary admitting diagnosis, condition before study of cause of inpatient admission
RAI: resident assessment instrument used in completing MDS in long-term care
RAP: resident assessment protocols used in completing MDS in long-term care
retrospective review: review of medical record after complete hospital stay; utilization function
risk management: the process of making and carrying out decisions that will minimize the adverse effects of accidental losses upon an organization
Senic Study on the Efficacy of Nosocomial Infection Control: study of infection control programs 1974-1984
severity of illness/intensity of service (SI/IS): documentation of clinical findings and prescribed medical care
surveillance: a procedure used to monitor and control infectious disease
surveillance by objective (SBO): different surveillance systems designed to monitor and control various types of infections
TEFRA: Tax Equity Fiscal Responsibility Act
utilization review: the assessment of the use of professional care, service, procedures, and evaluation of need and appropriateness of care
voluntary organizations: financed through private organizations and third-party payors

APPENDIX

A

Integrated Quality Management Tools

This appendix contains sample tools for ongoing monitoring and evaluation of the integrated quality management processes in nursing practice. These tools are designed for use in acute care but are adaptable to any health care setting.

PATIENT DAILY INTEGRATED QUALITY MANAGEMENT ASSESSMENT TOOL

This tool can be used by the primary nurse on a daily basis to monitor and evaluate the integrated quality management processes (Fig. A-1). It includes the patient's initials, medical record number, diagnosis/DRG, unit, and date of each assessment. Data can be used for patient care planning and intervention. It is not a permanent part of the medical record but should be retained for analysis and trending as part of quality assessment and improvement data collection.

UNIT DAILY INTEGRATED QUALITY MANAGEMENT ASSESSMENT TOOL

This tool is useful to the nurse manager on each unit to monitor and evaluate integrated quality management processes for all patients (Fig. A-2). It includes the patient's initials and room number with comments and outcomes for each patient. It provides a quick overview of any quality man-

Confidential

Patient's Initials: _____ Medical Record No. _____

Unit _____ Diagnosis/DRG _____ Expected LOS _____

Patient Daily Integrated Quality Management Assessment Tool*

Date	IC	RM/S	UM	QA/I	Comments/Outcome

*To be completed each day by the patient's primary nurse and included in continued assessment, planning, and intervention. Not a part of permanent record. Retain with QA/I data collection and analyze for trends.

FIGURE A-1
Patient daily integrated quality management assessment tool.

Confidential

Date _____   Unit _____

Unit Daily Integrated Quality Management Assessment Tool*

Patient Initials/Room No.	IC	RM/S	UM	QA/I	Comments/Outcome

*To be completed each day by the nurse manager for continuing assessment and intervention to improve patient outcomes. Not a part of permanent record. Retain with QA/I data collection and analyze for trends.

FIGURE A-2
Unit daily integrated quality management assessment tool.

agement concerns for the unit that day. The tool is not a permanent part of the medical record but is retained with quality assessment and improvement data collection for analysis and trending.

QUALITY MANAGEMENT CASE MANAGEMENT TOOL

This tool provides a summary of the patient's case with specific emphasis on each quality management process assessment and action plan (Fig. A-3). The case management conference tool provides a comprehensive summary of critical path/care track variance, as well as evaluation for continued monitoring and evaluation. The next conference date is included.

It gives the basic format for a QM case management conference and recording of pertinent data. The form is usually retained as part of the quality assessment and improvement data collection for trending and analysis.

QUALITY MANAGEMENT AGGREGATE VARIANCE ANALYSIS/TREND REPORT

The information from the Daily Patient and Unit QM Assessment Tools, as well as the QM Case Management Report, can provide data for this tool, which is a general analysis and trend report that is completed at specific time frames (monthly, quarterly) (Fig. A-4). It is useful in retrospective review and proactive planning for positive patient outcomes on a given unit or on various units. It is part of the monitoring and evaluation process for ongoing quality assessment and improvement in aggregate form.

Confidential
Quality Management Case Management Conference

Patient Initials _____ Date _____

Diagnosis/DRG _____ Unit _____

Medical Record No. _____

Critical Path/Care Track Variance:
_____
_____
_____

Brief case assessment and plan for each quality management area:

Infection Control:
_____
_____

Plan: _____

Risk Management/Safety:
_____
_____

Plan: _____

Utilization Management:
_____
_____

Plan: _____

Quality Assessment/Improvement:
_____
_____

Monitoring and Evaluation: _____

Evaluation and Summary:
_____
_____
_____
_____

Next Conference Review Date: _____

FIGURE A-3
Quality management case management tool.

Confidential
Quality Management Aggregate Varance Analysis/Trend Report

Unit _____   Date _____

Diagnosis/DRG _____

Number of Cases Reviewed _____

Time Frame/Period Covered _____

Quality Management Variances

Infection Control: Number of Cases _____
Action Taken: _____
Outcomes: _____

Risk/Safety Management: Number of Cases _____
Action Taken: _____
Outcomes: _____

Utilization Management: Number of Cases _____
Action Taken: _____
Outcomes: _____

Quality Assessment: Number of Cases _____
Action Taken: _____
Outcomes: _____

Monitor/Evaluation Planned:

Summary/Comments:

Completed by: _____

FIGURE A-4
Quality management aggregate variance analysis/trend report.

APPENDIX B

Case Studies

The following case studies demonstrate the proactive planning process for patients in various settings, using the integrated QM model. The "fishbone" cause-and-effect diagram described in Chapter 9 is used in each scenario.

This proactive process analyzes the possible root causes to produce a positive patient care outcome in each case. The cause-and-effect diagrams are best developed through a "brainstorming" session with several knowledgeable health care professionals. The possible root causes are defined in this model as issues related to infection control, risk/safety management, utilization management, and quality assessment and improvement. The desired goal is a positive patient outcome.

The fishbone diagram can be used to assess an adverse outcome as well. An example is a patient fall. After the fact, the nurse can assess the possible causes leading to the fall, such as poor lighting, medication side effects, improper footware, lack of staff availability, or patient weakness, as well as the impact on the other quality management processes. This retrospective analysis can then be the basis of proactive care planning to prevent future falls.

Fishbone diagrams can be developed as guidelines in planning care to address the general patient health care needs of any setting's scope of practice. The nurse can then individualize the appropriate diagram to the specific patient. The examples given are guidelines for a variety of settings from acute care to home care. They are representative of common cases nurses may encounter in the described setting. The goal is ongoing, proactive care planning that produces positive patient care outcomes in appropriate, safe environments.

CASE STUDY: ACUTE CARE

Mr. M. is a 72-year-old black male admitted to the hospital for abdominal pain, rectal bleeding, and dehydration (Fig. B-1). Further tests showed a large colon tumor. The biopsy was malignant. The internal medicine MD has called in a surgeon for bowel resection and possible colostomy.

The patient's daughter, Susan, accompanied him to the emergency room. She states her father has lost his appetite and consequently has lost weight. She tells the nurse that Mr. M.'s grandfather died from colon cancer, which he is reluctant to discuss. Mr. M. has a history of ulcerative colitis.

Susan explained that she has been his only care giver since her mother died from congestive heart failure a year ago. She lives only a mile from her father but cares for her two teenage children and works part time as well. Her home is small, but she would like to care for her father there, if possible.

CASE STUDY: OUTPATIENT SURGERY

Mrs. W. is a 72-year-old female who lives independently in her own home (Fig. B-2). She came to the outpatient surgery center for minor surgery. When marked fluctuations in her vital signs occurred after surgery, the physician decided to put her in an observation status bed for the remainder of the evening. Mrs. W. expected to go home the next morning.

The nurse gave Mrs. W. a sedative that night for sleep. During the night, Mrs. W. awoke and went to the bathroom. She slipped and fell in the bathroom, sustaining a fractured hip. Mrs. W. was then admitted to the hospital, where she has been for 2 weeks. The nursing staff in the outpatient surgery unit used the cause-and-effect diagram to assess all possible causes of Mrs. W.'s fall to plan proactively to prevent such occurrences in the future. This assessment was passed on to the unit where Mrs. W. was transferred for further development.

CASE STUDY: HOME CARE

Mr. N. is a 55-year-old white male who retired early from a lucrative law practice because of a debilitating stroke (Fig. B-3). He has a history of hypertension and workaholic behavior. He has been in a rehabilitation center and has now returned home for continued support.

He is overweight and has been unable to care for himself since the
(continued on page 239).

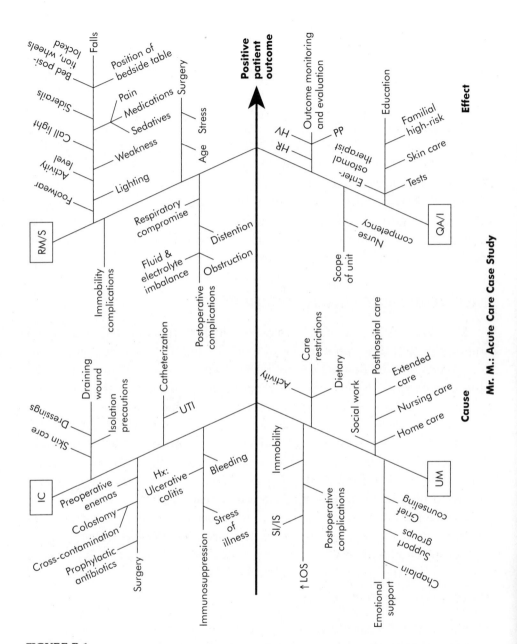

FIGURE B-1
Integrated quality management "fishbone" diagram: acute care case study. *IC*, infection control; *UM*, utilization management; *RM/S*, risk management/safety; *QA/I*, quality assessment/improvement; *HV*, high volume; *HR*, high risk; *PP*, problem prone.

APPENDIXES   237

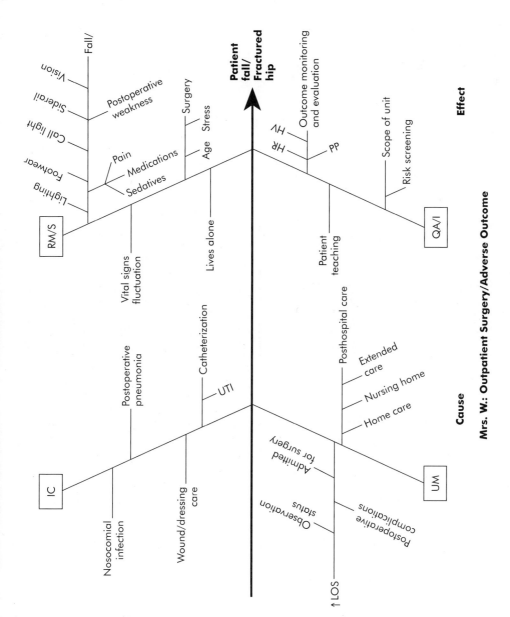

FIGURE B-2
Integrated quality management "fishbone" diagram: outpatient surgery case study. *IC*, infection control; *UM*, utilization management; *RM/S*, risk management/safety; *QA/I*, quality assessment/improvement; *HV*, high volume; *HR*, high risk; *PP*, problem prone.

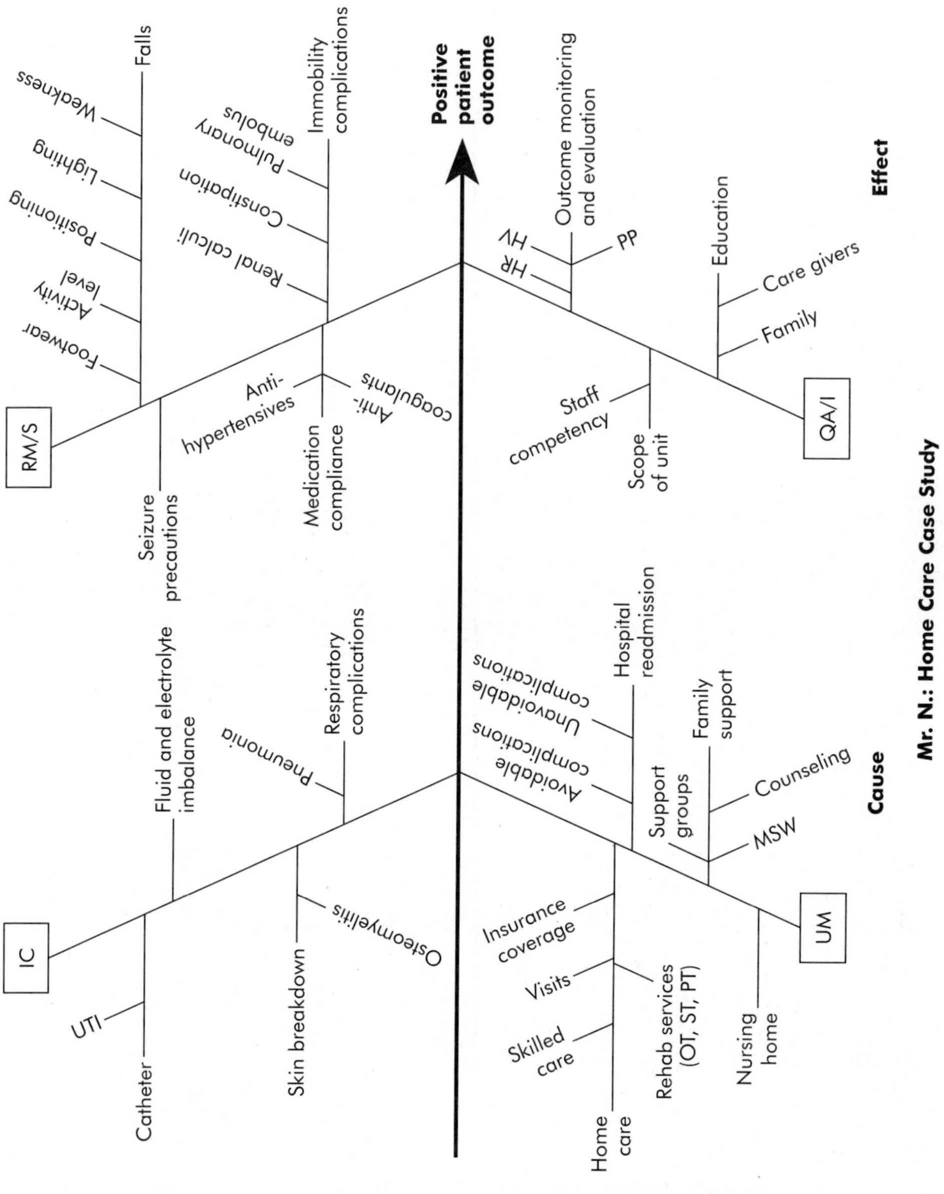

FIGURE B-3
Integrated quality management "fishbone" diagram: home care case study. *IC*, infection control; *UM*, utilization management; *RM/S*, risk management/safety; *QA/I*, quality assessment/improvement; *HV*, high volume; *HR*, high risk; *PP*, problem prone.

cardiovascular accident. He has several children in town, including a son who is a nurse at a local hospital. His wife employs an attendant from 10 PM to 6 AM each day to care for Mr. N. She also has a housekeeper who is available for light assistance to Mr. N. during the day. There is good family support. Mr. N.'s private insurance covers intermittent visits by a home care nurse each week.

CASE STUDY: AMBULATORY CARE

Mr. L. is a 63-year-old white male who comes to the ambulatory care center for an incision and drainage of a puncture wound in the lower right leg (Fig. B-4). He was gardening on his small field in a rural area several days ago when a stick punctured his leg. He put some salve on it, but it began to swell and throb with pain. He decided to go to the doctor when he started having a fever and had difficulty bearing weight on that leg.

Mr. L. gave a verbal history indicating that he lives with his 62-year-old wife who has severe arthritis and recently began chemotherapy for cancer. Mr. L. is the primary care giver and is dependent on a small pension and his garden produce. Mr. L. took early retirement because of progressive peripheral vascular disease.

CASE STUDY: LONG-TERM CARE

Mrs. B. is an 80-year-old female who lived independently in an older adult residence until several weeks ago (Fig. B-5). On the way to her mailbox, Mrs. B. slipped and fell, sustaining a hip fracture. Her neighbor called an ambulance, and Mrs. B. was taken to the hospital. She has now been transferred to a skilled nursing unit.

Mrs. B. is mentally alert and had been very active in her local community before the fall. She has two children and four grandchildren. The closest relative is her daughter who lives about 100 miles away. She has Medicare and a supplemental insurance policy. Her husband died approximately 5 years ago.

Mrs. B. has adult-onset diabetes, which is generally well controlled. She has a tendency toward hypoglycemia. She is insulin dependent and complies most of the time with dietary restrictions. She developed a small ulcer on her lower leg before hospitalization. Mrs. B. has poor vision and very fragile skin.

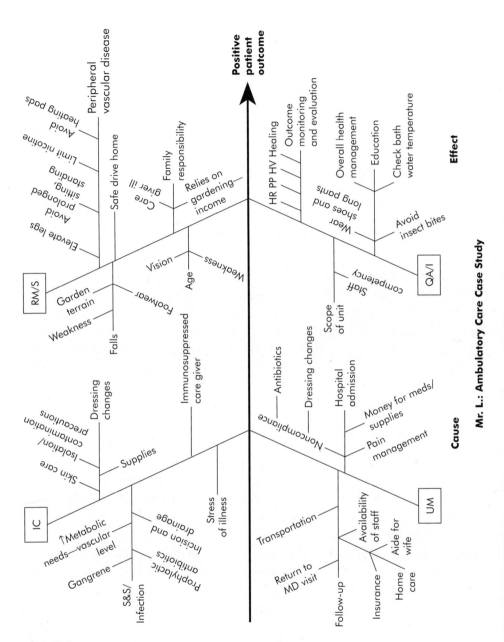

FIGURE B-4
Integrated quality management "fishbone" diagram: ambulatory care case study. *IC*, infection control; *UM*, utilization management; *RM/S*, risk management/safety; *QA/I*, quality assessment/improvement; *HV*, high volume; *HR*, high risk; *PP*, problem prone.

APPENDIXES 241

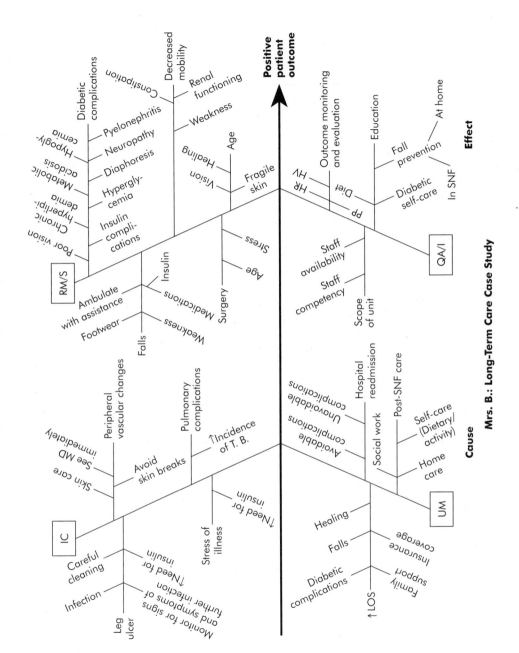

FIGURE B-5
Integrated quality management "fishbone" diagram: long-term care case study. *IC,* infection control; *UM,* utilization management; *RM/S,* risk management/safety; *QA/I,* quality assessment/improvement; *HV,* high volume; *HR,* high risk; *PP,* problem prone.

APPENDIX C

National Demonstration Project on Quality Improvement in Health Care

In 1987 the John A. Hartford Foundation sponsored the National Demonstration Project on Quality Improvement in Health Care (NDP). Twenty-one U.S. health care organizations were paired with quality experts from major U.S. companies, with improvement of health care services being the goal.

The NDP used many tools commonly found in industry to apply the theories and techniques of quality control to health care settings. These tools facilitate quality improvement. Fig. C-1 lists the quality improvement tools used in various steps of problem solving by the NDP.

Participants in this project included the following[*]:

HEALTH CARE ORGANIZATIONS

Beth Israel Hospital
Priscilla Dasse
Assistant Director

Peggy Reiley, RN, MS
Director of Quality Assurance and
  Development

Brigham & Women's Hospital
David Blumenthal, MD
Senior Vice President

Sheridan Kassirer
Vice President for Clinical Services
(continued on p. 244).

---

[*]From Berwick DM, Godfrey AB, Roessner J: *Curing health care: new strategies for quality improvement*, San Francisco, 1990, Jossey-Bass, pp 167–175.

Steps in problem solving		Quality Improvement Tools									
		Flow diagrams	Brainstorming	Cause-Effect diagrams	Data collection	Graphs and charts	Stratification	Pareto analysis	Histograms	Scatter diagrams	Control charts
Defining the Problem	1. List and prioritize problems	○	○		●	○	○	●			
	2. Define project and team	○				○	○				
The Diagnostic Journey	3. Analyze symptoms	●		●	○	○	●	○		○	
	4. Formulate theories of causes	○	●	●			○				
	5. Test theories	●			●	●	●	●	●	●	●
	6. Identify root causes	●			●	●	●	●	●	●	●
The Remedial Journey	7. Consider alternative solutions	●	●	○			○				
	8. Design solutions and controls	●			●	●	○		○	●	●
	9. Address resistance to change	○	●	○							
	10. Implement solutions and controls	●				○		○	○	○	
Holding the Gains	11. Check performance	○			●	●	●	●	●	○	●
	12. Monitor control system	○			●	●	●		○		●

Legend: ● Primary or frequent application of tool   ○ Secondary, infrequent, or circumstantial   ☐ None or very rare

FIGURE C-1
Applications for quality improvement tools. (From Berwick DM, Godfrey AB, Roessner J: *Curing health care: new strategies for quality improvement*, San Francisco, 1990, Jossey-Bass, p 179.)

Glenn Laffel, MD
Director, Quality Assurance Planning

H. Richard Nesson, MD
President

Butterworth Hospital

Randall Kehr
Department Manager, Respiratory Care

Randall J. Wagner
Vice President, Operations

The Children's Hospital

Robert K. Crone, MD
Director, Multidisciplinary ICU

David G. Nathan, MD
Chairman, Department of Medicine

The Evanston Hospital

Mark Neaman
President and COO

James Roberts, MD
Senior Vice President for Research and Planning

Joint Commission on Accreditation of Health Care Organizations

Dale Sowders
Assistant to the President

Group Health Cooperative of Puget Sound

Bruce Perry, MD, MPH
Director, Quality of Care Assessment

Cheryl M. Scott
Regional Vice President/Assistant COO

Harvard Community Health Plan

Stephen Baer, MD
Chief, OB/GYN

David Chin MD
President, Health Centers Division

David Cochran, MD
Director, Boston Center

Debra Cookson
Project Coordinator, Quality-of-Care Management

Lawrence Gottlieb, MD
Director of Clinical Guidelines Program

Diana Parks Forbes, RN, NP
Wellesley OB/GYN

Kay M. Larholt
Statistical Specialist

Johns Hopkins Health System

Theodore M. King, MD, PhD
Vice President, Medical Affairs

Steven H. Lipstein
Director, Program Development and Marketing

L. Reuven Pasternak, MD
Anesthesiology and Critical Care Medicine

Kaiser-Permanente Medical Care Program

Robert Formanek, MD
Assistant Director of Quality

Leonard Rubin, MD
Director of Quality

Bruce J. Sams, Jr, MD
Executive Director

Maine Medical Center

F. Stephen Larned, MD
Vice President for Medical Affairs

James M. Thomas, MD
Director of Surgical Education

Massachusetts General Hospital

George P. Baker, Jr, MD
Associate General Director for Medical Affairs

Elizabeth Bradley
Administrative Fellow

William Kent
Administrative Fellow

John Mahoney
Associate Director of Fiscal Affairs

Ann Prestipino
Director of Patient Services

Massachusetts Respiratory Hospital

John A. Barmack
District Vice President
Hospital Corporation of America

Maureen A. Bisognano
Administrator
Massachusetts Respiratory Hospital

C. David Hardison, PhD
Director of Quality Information and Technology
Hospital Corporation of America

S. Douglas Smith
President
Hospital Corporation of America

*The Medical Center
University of California, San Francisco*

Mary Jane Allison
Assistant Director

William B. Kerr
Director

The North Carolina Memorial Hospital

Mary A. Beck
Director, Program and Planning Development

Eric B. Munson
Executive Director

Henriette (Hank) Neal
Associate Director of Operations

Park Nicollet Medical Center

James L. Reinertsen, MD
President

The Presbyterian Hospital in the City of New York

Patricia A. Chambers
Senior Administrator for Professional Affairs

Una Doddy
Administrative Resident for Medical Affairs

Thomas Q. Morris, MD
President & CEO

Gerald Thompson, MD
Executive Vice President for Professional Affairs

Rhode Island Group Health Association

Kathleen Malo
Operations Analyst

Richard Rosen, MD
Associate Medical Director

Strong Memorial Hospital, University of Rochester Medical Center

Leo P. Brideau
Director of Hospital Operations

Robert J. Panzer, MD
Associate Director of Quality
   Assurance

UCLA School of Medicine
Roberta Killingsworth
Deputy Director of Ambulatory
   Services
Neil H. Parker, MD
Director of Medical Ambulatory
   Services

University of Michigan Hospitals
Richard J. Coffey, PhD
Director, Management Systems
Deborah Hetland-Guglielmo
Associate Director of Nursing
Ellen J. Marszalek-Gaucher
Senior Associate Director
Mary Decker Staples
Associate Administrator

Worcester Memorial Hospital (since renamed *The Med Center Memorial Hospital*)
Harry G. Dorman, III
Executive Vice President/COO
Laurence E. Kelly
Vice President, Professional Services

QUALITY ADVISERS

Professor David Bush
Department of Psychology
Villanova University

Haggai Cohen
Formerly with NASA

Christie E. Cook, PhD
Behavioral Health Services
CIGNA

J. Douglas Ekings
Manager, Customer Satisfaction
Xerox Corporation

Allen C. Endres, PhD
Vice President
Juran Institute, Inc.

Mary Ann Gould
President
Total Quality Management
   Association

David Groff, PhD
Director of Manager/Management
   Training
Corning Glass Works

Berton H. Gunter
Statistical Consultant

David H. Gustafson, PhD
Department of Industrial Engineering
University of Wisconsin, Madison

Jeffrey H. Hooper, PhD
Quality Theory and Computing
   Group
AT&T Bell Laboratories

Robert W. Hungate
Director of Government Affairs
Hewlett-Packard

Robert King
Executive Director
GOAL

Professor Peter Kolesar
Graduate School of Business
Columbia University

Burton S. Liebesman, PhD
District Manager
Bell Communications Research

James Peterson
Manager, Employee Benefits
Florida Power and Light

Paul E. Plsek
President
Paul E. Plsek and Associates

James F. Riley, Jr.
Vice President
Juran Institute, Inc.
(formerly with IBM)

Professor Josef Schmee
Graduate Management Institute
Union College

Debra Shenk
Quality Manager
Hewlett-Packard Corporate Offices

Professor David Sylwester
Department of Statistics
University of Tennessee

Stephen A. Zayac, PhD
Ford Motor Co.

ADVISORY COMMITTEE

Paul B. Batalden, MD
Vice President for Medical Care
Hospital Corporation of America

Donald M. Berwick, MD
Vice President for Quality-of-Care
  Measurement
Harvard Community Health Plan

Howard S. Frazier, MD
Department of Health Policy and
  Management
Harvard School of Public Health

David A. Garvin, PhD
Professor of Business Administration
Harvard Business School

A. Blanton Godfrey, PhD
Chairman and CEO
Juran Institute, Inc.

David H. Gustafson, PhD
Chairman, Department of Industrial
  Engineering
University of Wisconsin, Madison

David Hemenway, PhD
Assistant Professor of Political
  Economy
Harvard School of Public Health

Marian Knapp
Director, Quality-of-Care
  Measurement
Harvard Community Health Plan

Ellen J. Marszalek-Gaucher
Senior Associate Director
University of Michigan Hospitals

Lincoln Moses, PhD
Department of Statistics
Stanford University

Frederick Mosteller, PhD
Department of Health Policy and
  Management
Harvard School of Public Health

R. Heather Palmer, MB, BCh, SM
Department of Health Policy and
  Management
Harvard School of Public Health

Mitchell T. Rabkin, MD
President
Beth Israel Hospital

James Roberts, MD
Senior Vice President for Research
  and Planning
Joint Commission on Accreditation of
  Health Care Organizations

James Schlosser, MD
Clinical Director, National
  Demonstration Project
Harvard Community Health Plan

APPENDIX

D

Bibliography

Articles

Anderson CA, Daigh RD: Quality mind-set overcomes barriers to success, *Healthcare Financial Management* 45(2):20–22,24,26–32, 1991.

Appel F: From quality assurance to quality improvement: *The Joint Commission and the New Quality Paradigm* 13(5):26–29, 1991.

Berger S, Sudman SK: Making total quality management work, *Healthcare Executive* 6(2):22–25, 1991.

Berwick DM: Continuous quality improvement as an ideal in health care, *N Eng J Med* 320:53,56, 1989.

Burda D: Total quality management becomes big business, *Modern Healthcare* 21(4):25–29, 1991.

Bush D: Quality management through statistics, *J Qual Assur* 13(5):40–48, 1991.

Casalou RF: Total quality management in health care, *Hospital and Health Services Administration* 36(1):134–146, 1991.

Claflin N: Nursing QA in the '90s: revisions in the JCAHO nursing services standards, *J Qual Assur* 12(5):20–23, 1990.

Day G: Evaluating a nursing QA program, *J Qual Assur* 12(3):22–25, 1990.

Dimond FC Jr: What QA is and isn't. What TQM is and isn't. *QRC Advisor* 7(8):1–6, 1991.

Duncan RP, Fleming EC, Gallati TG: Implementing a continuous quality improvement program in a community hospital, *Qual Rev Bull* 17(4):106–112, 1991.

Ellison J, editor: How do QI, QA relate? Experts refute common myths, *Hospital Peer Review* 16(6):81–85, 1991.

Kazemek E, Peterson K: Hospitals must demonstrate commitment to total quality, *Healthcare Financial Management* 43(3):114,116, 1989.

Koska MT: Adopting Deming's quality improvement ideas: a case study, *Hospitals* 64(13):58–64, 1990.

Labavitz, GH: Beyond the total quality mystique, *Healthcare Executive* 6(2):15–17, 1991.
Naehring M: The nursing process: watching it happen at Woodland Memorial Hospital, *J Qual Assur* 13(2):20–24, 1991.
O'Leary DS: Accreditation in the quality improvement mold—a vision for tomorrow, *Joint Commission Perspectives* 10(2):2–3, 1990.
Puta DF: Nurse-physician collaboration toward quality, *J Nurs Qual Assur* 3(2):11–17, 1989.
Roster SL: Total quality improvement, *J Qual Assur* 12(4):18–21, 1990.
Sinioris ME: TQM: the new frontier for quality and productivity improvement in health care, *J Qual Assur* 12(4):14–17.
Williams T, Howe R: W. Edwards Deming and total quality management: an interpretation for nursing practice, *J Healthcare Qual* 14(1):36–39, 1992.

Books

Avillion AE, Mirgon B: *Quality assurance in rehabilitation nursing: a practical guide*, Frederick, Calif, 1989, Aspen Publishers.
Balau J: *Quality assurance policies and procedures for home health care*, Frederick, Calif, 1989, Aspen Publishers.
Berwick DM, Godfrey AB, Roessner J: *Curing health care: new strategies for quality improvement*, San Francisco, 1990, Jossey-Bass.
Block P: *The empowered manager*, San Diego, 1990, University Associates.
Boschon S: *A complete guide to utilization management*, Fayetteville, NC, 1990, Continuing Education Resources, Publications Department.
Bush DL: *Quality improvement in health care organizations*, Blackwood, NJ, 1991, Diversified Business Associates.
Congress of the United States Office of Technology Assessment: *The quality of medical care: information for consumers*, 1988, Washington, DC.
Crosby PB: *Let's talk quality*, New York, 1989, McGraw-Hill.
Crosby PB: *Quality is free*, New York, 1979, New American Library.
InterQual: *A guide to clinical risk management*, North Hampton, NH, 1990.
James BC: *Quality management for health care delivery*, Chicago, 1989, American Hospital Association.
Johnson M, editor: *The delivery of quality health care, series on nursing administration*, vol 3 St. Louis, March 1992, Mosby–Year Book.
Juran JM: *Juran on leadership for quality*, New York, 1989, Free Press.
Juran JM: *Juran on planning for quality*, New York, 1988, Free Press.
Katz J, Green E: *Managing quality: a guide to monitoring and evaluating nursing services*, St. Louis, 1992, Mosby–Year Book.
Leebov, W: *The quality quest: a briefing for health care professionals*, Chicago, 1991, American Hospital Publishing.

Marszalek-Gaucher E, Coffey R: *Transforming health care organizations: how to achieve and sustain organizational excellence*, San Francisco, 1990, Jossey-Bass.

Rowland H, Rowland B: *Manual of nursing quality assurance*, Frederick, Md, 1987, 1989, Aspen Publishers.

Spath PL: *Health care quality: a practical guide to continuous improvement*, Portland, Ore, 1991, Brown-Soath Associates.

Walton M: *The Deming management method*, Putnam, NY, 1986, Dodd, Mead & Co.

Williams T, Howe R: *Applying total quality management: a nursing guide*, Chicago, 1991, Precept Press.

Journals

Healthcare Forum Journal. The Healthcare Forum, 830 Market Street, San Francisco, 94102 (415) 421-8810.

Bimonthly, features articles on issues in quality management and leadership.

Health Law Trends. Arent Fox Kintner Plotkin & Kahn, 1050 Connecticut Ave, NW, Washington, DC, 20036-5339 (202) 857-6000.

Hospital Peer Review. American Health Consultants, 67 Peachtree Park Drive, NE, Atlanta, 30309-1937 (800) 554-1032.

Monthly, features current issues in hospital quality management, including utilization management, PRO, and discharge planning.

Joint Commission Perspectives. One Renaissance Blvd, Oakbrook Terrace, Ill, 60181 (708) 916-5600.

Bimonthly newsletter, keeps health care organizations updated on changes in accreditation standards, scoring guidelines, and Agenda for Change. Offers practical tips on how to meet compliance; includes examples.

Journal for Healthcare Quality (Formerly, Journal of Quality Assurance) National Association for Healthcare Quality. 5700 Old Orchard Road, First Floor, Skokie, Ill, 60077-1057 (708) 966-9392.

Bimonthly, by professionals for professionals in all areas of healthcare quality. Addresses quality assessment and improvement, risk management, utilization management, managed care, JCAHO, PRO, data collection and analysis, and other areas. Submissions published earns CEU credits for retaining status as certified professional in healthcare quality.

Nursing Quality Connection. Mosby–Year Book, 11830 Westline Industrial Drive, St. Louis, 63146 (800) 325-4177.

Outcomes, Measurement & Management. The Center for Outcome Measurement, 605 Market Street, Suite 1111, San Francisco, 94105 (415) 495-2450.

Bimonthly newsletter published through an educational grant by Syntex. Devoted to health care outcomes and cost-effectiveness issues.

QI/TQM. American Health Consultants, 67 Peachtree Park Drive, NE Atlanta, 30309-1937 (800) 554-1032.

Monthly newsletter with practical applications for quality improvement.

The Quality Letter for Healthcare Leaders. Bader & Associates, Inc., PO Box 2106, Rockville, Md, 20852 (310) 468-1610.

Newsletter for senior management for monitoring trends and strategies for quality management.

Quality Management Update. Care Communications, 101 E. Ontario, Chicago, 60611 (312) 943-0463.

Monthly newsletter, information on quality improvement/quality management, JCAHO, conference locations.

Quality, Risk, and Cost Advisor. Aspen Publishers, 7201 McKinney Circle, Frederick, Md, 21701 (800) 638-8437.

Monthly newsletter, addresses quality, utilization, and risk management.

Catalogs

Joint Commission on Accreditation of Healthcare Organizations: 1992 Publications Catalog. One Renaissance Boulevard, Oakbrook Terrace, Ill, 60181 (708) 916-5600, 7 AM–5 PM Central Standard Time.

Audiocassettes, accreditation manuals and scoring guidelines, examples of monitoring and evaluation, periodicals, plant, technology, and safety management, quality improvement, videocassettes.

JCAHO Blue Book Directory (708) 916-5600.

A directory to facilitate better communication with JCAHO. Has a PhoneMail system. Fax number of JCAHO is (708) 916-5645. Includes an organizational chart, divisions, and departments, with functions and phone extensions. Also has a one-page fact sheet on JCAHO.

Videotapes

Kaisen: Continuous Quality Improvement: A Blueprint for Outcome Measures. CHAP, 350 Hudson Street, New York, NY 10014 (212) 989-9393 Fax (212) 989-3710.

A 40-minute video approved for 0.2 CED's by the NLN.

Total Quality Management: Ten Elements for Implementing. Goal QPC, 13 Branch Street, Methuen, Mass, 10844 (508) 685-6370.

Ten videotapes ranging from 9 to 23 minutes in length on subjects such as understanding the customer, initial pilot project teams, managing TQM momentum, new functional and cross functional teams, and reviewing the 5 year plan with TQM.

Index

A

Accountability, interdisciplinary collaborative practice and, 140
Acute care, 158–167
  case study on, 235, *236*
  continuous quality improvement in, 166–167
  hospitals for, history of, 158–159
  quality management in
    case examples of, 163–166
    integrated, 131–132
    clinical, 161–167
    in management
      of congestive heart failure patient, 163–164
      of diabetic patient, 164–166
    Peer Review Organization in, 161–163
    unique issues in, 160–161
  in 1990s, 159–160
Administrative concerns, utilization management and, 88–89
Advisors, quality, in National Demonstration Project on quality improvement in health care, 246–247
Advisory committee in National Demonstration Project on quality improvement in health care, 247
Aging, factor influencing, 196–197
Ambulatory care, case study on, 239, *240*
Ambulatory care services, scope of care in, 71
Ambulatory care setting, 168–170
  cancer care services in, 172–173
  cardiovascular services in, 173
  clinical laboratory services in, 172
  emergency services in, 171
  freestanding, 169
  health care services available in, 170–174

Ambulatory care setting–cont'd
  high-technology diagnostic imaging and radiology in, 171–172
  hospital-based, 168–169
  outpatient surgery in, 170–171
  physician office-based, 169–170
  quality improvement in, National Demonstration Project on, 181–182
  quality management clinical indicators in, 179–180
  rehabilitation services in, 173
  unique issues in, 174–175

B

Bioethics, 214
Business
  definitions of terms in, 24
  Japanese vs. Western quality control in, 33–34
  leaders in quality improvement in, 24–33
  quality assessment in, 34–35
  quality improvement in, 35
    six steps to, 35–37
  total quality control in history of, 22–23

C

Cancer care services in ambulatory care setting, 172–173
Cardiovascular ambulatory services, 173
Case management in utilization management, 85
Case studies, 234–241
Cause-and-effect diagram as quality management tool, 125–128
Centers for Disease Control (CDC), creation of, 113
CHAMPUS insurance, 49–50
Client satisfaction, quality management and, 7

Clients, risks to, 99–100
Clinical laboratory ambulatory services, 172
Collaborative, definition of, 139
Collaborative practice
  benefits to nursing and patient care from, 142–143
  definition of, 139–140
  examples of, 144–148
  in implementing quality improvement teams, 148–150
  interdisciplinary, factors promoting/hindering, 140–142
  introduction to, 138
  strategies for, 143–144
Communication, interdisciplinary collaborative practice and, 140, 141–142
Competence, interdisciplinary collaborative practice and, 140
Comprehensive Older Americans Act, 198
Computerization in future of quality management, 219–220
Confidentiality of quality assessment activities, 67
Congestive heart failure, clinical quality management of, 163–164
Consumerism, quality management and, 7
Continuous quality improvement (CQI)
  in acute care services, 166–167
  in home health care, 188–189
  infection control and, 117
  resident assessment instrument of, in long-term care, 203–204
  utilization management and, 87–88
Cost containment era of 1970s, 47–48
Crosby, Philip B., on quality management, 31–33

D

Deaths in acute care records review, 162
Decision making, interdisciplinary collaborative practice and, 141
Deming, W. Edwards
  on quality control programs, 24–28
  on quality management in health care, 40
Deming's Plan-Do-Check-Action (PDCA) approach to quality improvement, 35–37
Diabetic patient, clinical quality management of, 164–166

Diagnostic related groups (DRGs)
  pricing based on, 48, 49
  prospective pricing system based on, 77
Differences, valued, 16
Discharge planning
  adequacy of, in acute care records review, 161
  utilization management and, 85
Donabedian, Avedis, on quality management in health care, 39–40
Drug errors, eliminating, in acute care services, 166–167
Drugs, utilization of, in long-term care facilities, OBRA and, 200–201

E

Education in safety programs, 104
Elderly, legislation and organizations to aid, 197–200
Emergency services
  in ambulatory care setting, 171
  scope of care in, 71–72
Enforcement in safety programs, 104
Engineering in safety programs, 104
Epidemiology, 113–114
Ethics in future of quality management, 214–217

F

Fiscal intermediary relationship, home health care and, 188
Fishbone cause-and-effect diagram in case studies, 234, 236–238, 240–241
Freestanding ambulatory care, 169
Future of quality management, 209–223
  ethics in, 214–217
  high technology in, 218–220
  integrated, 223
  marketing in, 220–221
  nursing agenda for health care reform in, 222–223
  research in, 209–214
  supplemental staffing agencies in, 222
  third-party review and payors in, 217–218

G

"Gag Rule," 215–216
General public, risks to, 100–101
Generic quality screens
  for hospital outpatient department, 178–179
  for outpatient surgery, 177

G

Government
  response of, to malpractice crisis, 92
  support for health care expansion by, 46, 47

H

Health care
  managed, 51–53
  quality improvement in, National Demonstration Project on, 41–42
  quality management in, 37–42
    history of quality review in, 37–39
    industrial models applied to, 40–41
    leaders in, 37–39
  safety in, 105–106, 107–108
Health care employer, risks to, 98–99
Health Care Financing Administration (HCFA), 48
Health care organizations in National Demonstration Project on quality improvement in health care, 242, 244–246
Health insurance, history of, 44–46
Health Maintenance Organizations (HMOs), 51–53
  home health care and, 187
High technology, home health care and, 186
High-technology diagnostic imaging and radiology in ambulatory care setting, 171
High technology in future of quality management, 218–220
HIV, mandatory testing and disclosure of, 216–217
Home care
  case study on, 235, *238*
  high-technology, 218–219
Home Care Quality Improvement (HCQI) Act, 76–77
Home health care, 184–194
  agencies for, types of, 187–188
  continuous quality improvement in, 188–189
  evolution of, 184–186
  fiscal intermediary relationship and, 188
  future of, 193
  high technology and, 186
  HMO/PPO use and, 187
  hospice movement and, 186–187
  implications of, for nursing, 194

Home health care–cont'd
  infection control in, 119, 192
  influences of, 184–186
  integrated quality management in, 134–135
  quality assessment in, 189–190
  risk management in, 190–191
  utilization management and, 192–193
Home health services, scope of care in, 72
Hospice movement in United States, 186–187
Hospital-based ambulatory care, 168–169

I

Illness, chronic, factors influencing, 196–197
Independent Practice Association (IPA), 52
Industrial safety growth and results of, 104
Industry
  quality assessment in, 34–35
  quality improvement systems in, 35
Infection(s), nosocomial
  in acute care records review, 162
  rates and types of, 115–116
Infection control, 19, 111–120
  administrative concerns on, 117
  for congestive heart failure patient, 164
  continuous quality improvement and, 117
  in diabetic patient, 165
  epidemiology and, 113–114
  future implications/benefits of, 117
  in home health care, 119, 192
  JCAHO and, 116
  in long-term care, 118–119, 205
  nursing and, 117
  scientific basis for, 114–115
  surveillance by objectives in, 116
Information management systems for ambulatory care, 175
Institutional long-term care, type of, 201–202
Insurance, health, history of, 44–46
Insurance companies, response of, to malpractice crisis, 92
Integrated quality management, 131–137
  in acute care, 131–132

Integrated quality management—cont'd
   in ambulatory care setting, 175–181
   future of, 223
   in home care, 134–135
   implications of, for professional
      nursing practice, 136–137
   in long-term care, 132–133
   in outpatient surgery, 135–136
   strategies for, 128–131
Integrated quality management model,
   123–128
Integrated quality management tool(s),
   228–233
   aggregate variance analysis/trend
      report as, 231, *234*
   assessment
      patient daily, 228, *229*
      unit daily, 228, *230*, 231
   case management, 231, *232*
Integration
   definition of, 121
   of quality management processes,
      122–123
   strategies for, 128–131
Interdisciplinary, definition of, 139–140

J

Japanese vs. Western quality control, 33–34
Joint Commission on Accreditation
   (JCOA), 49
Joint Commission on Accreditation of
   Health Care Organizations
   (JCAHO)
   in history of health care quality
      review, 37–39
   infection control and, 116
   monitoring and evaluation process of
      10-step, 60–66
   risk management and, 101–102
   safety standards and, 106–107
   standards of, 49–50
      on quality assurance, 57
   utilization management program and, 85
Juran, J. M., on product quality, 28–31

L

Leaders in quality improvement in
   business, 24–33
Legislation to aid elderly, 197–200
Liability claims
   increased underlying causes of, 92
   personal, rule of, 97

Life ethics, 214
Long-term care
   aging and, 196–197
   case study on, 239, *241*
   chronic illness and, 196–197
   CQI-resident assessment instrument
      in, 203–204
   implications of, for nursing practice,
      206
   infection control in, 118–119, 205
   institutional, types of, 201–202
   integrated quality management in,
      132–133
   legislation and organizations to aid
      elderly and, 197–200
   OBRA and drug utilization in,
      200–201
   quality assessment in, 202–203
   quality management in, 196–208
   risk management in, 205–206
   utilization management in, 205
Long-term care services, scope of care
   in, 72
Loss exposures, identifying and
   analyzing, 94–95

M

Malpractice, definition of, 97
Malpractice crisis
   government/insurance response to, 92
   second, 92
Managed care, 51–53
Management-directed success factors, *10*
Marketing in future of quality
   management, 220–221
Media emphasis quality management,
   6–7
Medicaid, elderly and, 198
Medical ethics, 214
Medical nursing, scope of care in, 70
Medical stability of patient in acute care
   records review, 162
Medicare, 46–47
   elderly and, 198
Minimum data set (MDS) for resident
   assessment, 199–200

N

National Demonstration Project (NDP)
   on quality improvement in health
   care, 41–42, 247–251
National response to staph pandemic, 113

National safety legislation on creation of OSHA, 104–105
Natural synergy, 13–14
Negligence, definition of, 96–97
Neuman's system model, 123–125
Nosocomial infections
 in acute care records review, 162
 rates and types of, 115–116
Nurse professional, individual risks for, 97–98
Nursing
 administrative implications of quality management for, 9
 agenda of, for health care reform in future of quality management, 222–223
 benefits of collaborative practice to, 142–143
 infection control and, 118
 risk management process in, 95–96
 roles and responsibilities of, quality assessment/improvement process in, 59
 safety in, 107–108
Nursing practice
 defining scope of, in each nursing area, 68
 implications for
  of home health care, 194
  of quality assessment/improvement process, 67
  of quality management, 8–9
  of risk management, 109–110

O

Obstetric nursing, scope of care in, 71
Occupation Safety and Health Act (OSHA)
 creation of, national safety legislation on, 104–105
 regional programs of, 105
Older Americans Act, 197
Omnibus Budget Reconciliation Act (OBRA) of 1986, 199–200
 drug utilization in long-term care and, 200–201
 outpatient surgery and, 170
Operating room, scope of care in, 71
Organizational synergy, 15–16
Outpatient clinic in ambulatory care setting, integrated quality management in, 177–178

Outpatient invasive procedure documentation, 179
Outpatient surgery
 adverse outcome of, case study on, 235, 237
 in ambulatory care setting, 170–171
 integrated quality management in, 176–177
 integrated quality management in, 135–136
Overutilization of resources in utilization management, 86

P

Patient care, benefits of collaborative practice to, 142–143
Patient classification systems in utilization management, 82–83
Patient daily integrated quality management assessment tool, 228, 229
Patients, risks to, 99–100
Peer Review Organization (PRO), 50–51
 in acute care setting, 161–163
 enforcement mechanisms of, 77
 responsibilities of, to Health Care Financing Administration, 74–75
 review of, Title VI Social Security Amendment and, 75–76
Physician office-based ambulatory care, 169–170
Preferred Provider Organizations (PPOs), 52
 home health care and, 187
Processes of quality management, 12–21; see also Synergy
Productivity evaluations for ambulatory care, 174–175
Psychiatric services, scope of care in, 72
Public, general, risks to, 100–101

Q

Quality
 in ambulatory care, 175
 of life, 202
Quality advisors in National Demonstration Project on quality improvement in health care, 246–247
Quality assessment
 activities of, confidentiality of, 67
 of congestive heart failure patient, 163–164

Quality assessment—cont'd
  of diabetic patient, 164–168
  in home health care, 189–190
  and improvement (QA/QI), 17
  in industry, 34–35
  in long-term care, 202–203
  utilization management and, 85–86
Quality assessment/improvement process
  development of, 59
  implications of, for practice, 67
  in nursing roles and responsibilities, 59
Quality assurance
  definition of, 56
  history of, 57
  versus quality improvement, 57–58
Quality control
  definition of, 24
  Japanese vs. Western, 33–34
  total, in business history of, 22–23
Quality improvement
  definition, 56
  in health care, National Demonstration Project on, 242–251
  history of, 57
  versus quality assurance, 57–58
Quality improvement systems in industry, 35
Quality improvement teams, implementing, 148–155
Quality management
  in business, 22–37; *see also* Business
  cause-and-effect diagram in, 125–128
  components of, 16–17
  consumerism and, 7
  definition of, 2–5
  future of, 209–223; *see also* Future of quality management
  goals of, 5–6
  in health care, 37–42; *see also* Health care
  implications of
    for collaborative practice, 138–156; *see also* Collaborative practice
    for nursing administration, 9
    for nursing practice, 8–9
  infection control and, 11–120; *see also* Infection control
  influences of, 6–8
  integration of components into, 3–5
  introduction to, 1–10
  media emphasis of, 6–7

Quality management—cont'd
  processes of, 12–21; *see also* Synergy
  integration of, 121–137; *see also* Integrated quality management
  regulation and, 7–8
  regulatory influences on, 44–55; *see also* Regulatory influences on quality management
  reimbursement and, 7, 8
  risk management in, 18
  safety/risk management in, 102
  synergy in, 12–21; *see also* Synergy
  utilization management in, 18–19
  valued differences in, 16
Quality management aggregate variance analysis/trend report, 231, 233
Quality management case management tool, 231, 232
Quality management clinical indicators in ambulatory care services, 179–180
Quality management synergy, 20

R
Regulation, quality management, 7–8
Regulatory influences on quality management, 44–55
  in CHAMPUS insurance, 49–50
  in government support for health care expansion, 46
  in health insurance, 44–46
  in managed care, 51–53
  Medicare and, 46–47
  in Peer Review Organization, 50–51
  in 1970s cost containment era, 47–48
  in 1980s policy shift, 48–49
  utilization management and, 53
Rehabilitation services, ambulatory, 172
Reimbursement
  for ambulatory care, 174
  quality management and, 7–8
Reimbursement/third-party payors in utilization management, 83–84
Research in future of quality management, 209–214
Resources, under/overutilization of, in utilization management, 86
"Right to Die," 214–215
Risk(s)
  to general public, 100–101
  health care, identification of, 96–101
  to health care employer, 98–99
  to individual nurse professional, 97–98
  to patient, client, or visitor, 99–100

Risk management, 18
  for congestive heart failure patient, 164
  definition of, 92–94
  for diabetic patient, 165
  emergence of, 91
  in home health care, 190–191
  implications of, for practice, 109–110
  introduction to, 90
  Joint Commission on Accreditation of Health Care Organizations and, 101–102
  in long-term care, 205–206
  loss exposure identification in, 94–95
  in outpatient surgery, 177
  process of, nursing and, 95–96
  in quality management, 102
  safety and, 90–111
Role conflict, interdisciplinary collaborative practice and, 141

S

Safety
  in health care, 105–106, 107–108
  implications of, for practice, 109–110
  industrial, growth and results of, 104
  in nursing, 107–108
  nursing implications/clinical concerns on, 109
  psychologic factors of, 107
  in quality management and; see also Risk management
  risk management and, 90–110
Safety Council creation of, 104
Safety hazards for health care workers, 108
Safety management
  for congestive heart failure patient, 164
  for diabetic patient, 165
Scientific basis for infection control, 114–115
Shewhart cycle, 22, 23
Social Security Act, Title VI, PRO review and, 75–76
Social synergy, 14–15
Special care unit, scope of care in, 72
Staffing agencies, supplemental, in future of quality management, 222–223
Staph pandemic, national response to, 113
Substance abuse services, scope of care in, 72

Surgery, unscheduled returns to, in acute care records review, 163
Surgical nursing, scope of care in, 70
Surveillance by objectives (SBO) in infection control, 116
Synergy
  characteristics of, 13
  natural, 13–14
  organizational, 15–16
  quality management, 20
  social, 14–15

T

Tax Equity and Fiscal Responsibility Act (TEFRA), 48, 74
Third-party review and payors in future of quality management, 217–218
Title VI Social Security Amendment, PRO review and, 75–76
Total quality control in business, history of, 22–23
Trauma suffered in hospital in acute care records review, 163

U

Underutilization of resources in utilization management, 86
Unit daily integrated quality management assessment tool, 228, 230
Utilization management, 18–19, 53, 73–78
  activities in, 79–80
  administrative concerns and, 88–89
  case management in, 84
  case mix in, 83
  for congestive heart failure patient, 164
  continuous quality improvement (CQI) and, 87–88
  criteria for, 81
  systems of, 81–82
  data in, management of, 82
  for diabetic patient, 165–166
  discharge planning in, 85
  examples of, in different settings, 86–87
  historical basis of, 73–78
  in home health care, 192–193
  Joint Commission of, 85
  in long-term care, 205
  in outpatient surgery, 176–177
  patient classification systems in, 82–83

Utilization management—cont'd
  program for, creation of, 78
  quality assessment and, 85–86
  reimbursement/third-party payors in, 83–84
  review in, approaches to, 80
  under/overutilization of resources in, 86

V
Valued differences, 16
Visitors, risks to, 99–100

W
Western vs. Japanese quality control, 33–34
White House Conferences on Aging, 197
Workman's compensation programs in United States, evolution of, 102–103